A Taste of the Good Life

A Cookbook for an Interstitial Cystitis Diet

▲ ▲ ▲

by Beverley Laumann

A Taste of the Good Life: A Cookbook for an Interstitial Cystitis Diet

Publisher:
Freeman Family Trust Publications
P.O. Box 402
Tustin, CA 92781

Printer:
KNI Inc.

Cover design, illustrations & graphics
Beverley Laumann

First edition
published 1998
printed in the United States

ISBN 0-9665706-0-X
Library of Congress Catalog Card Number: 98-73062

CONTENTS

PART TWO

PREFACE

As anyone with IC knows, pain and exhaustion can take a toll on even the most determined. We struggle with details of daily living that most people take for granted. With time though, many of us learn to accommodate our medical condition, cope with the day-to-day difficulties, and approach life with renewed enthusiasm, new priorities, and a positive outlook.

In large part, making that adjustment involves the discovery that one is not alone in struggling with interstitial cystitis. We all need to feel connected, to feel a part of something, even though the disease itself tends to isolate us. Finding and talking to others with IC has been for me, a way to fight back, and in hearing their stories, I feel connected. There is something very deeply moving and precious— healing even— about finding others who have experienced what we have experienced, first hand.

My IC story

Each of us with IC has our own IC "story," our take on how we got where we are. Many of us had chronic bladder infections or surgery shortly before we began to experience the IC. Each of us wonders if it was something we did that brought this on. Some of us have had the blessing of symptom-free remissions, lasting months or years. This is not unusual when we first get the disease. But for all of us, though we are relieved to finally have a label for our problem, being told the diagnosis is interstitial cystitis can be emotionally devastating. We all go through an emotional low point following diagnosis, as the words "chronic" and "incurable" sink in. It can be just as traumatic as losing a loved one or going through divorce.

Though I occasionally had urinary tract infections at various times throughout my life, my bladder trouble turned serious back in 1984. I was a young mother, in my early thirties, staying home to enjoy raising my two young children. In the fall of that year I came down with the flu, which quickly turned into a case of bronchitis. While I was on antibiotics for the bronchitis, I developed an excruciating bladder infection. My doctor switched antibiotics to clear up the bladder infection, but few weeks later another bladder infection set in. Within a short time, bladder infections became a monthly occurrence. Though the bladder infections would initially go away when faced with an onslaught of antibiotics, eventually they didn't seem to respond.

Finally in the summer of 1986, after two years of bladder pain, my urologist hinted at interstitial cystitis as an explanation. He wanted to do a cystoscopy in the hospital to take a good look at my bladder. I told him I'd think about it. By this time I was developing some severe pollen allergies, too. Weeks passed. While I was still mulling his comments over, the bladder symptoms suddenly disappeared. No more urethral burning, no more running to the bathroom every few minutes, no more infections. "Aha," I thought, "he was wrong! It's not IC! I'm cured!"

For the next couple of years I felt totally healthy, although I was still bothered by seasonal allergies. Then, just as suddenly as the bladder pain had disappeared, it was back in my life again. With it came a deep abdominal pain I hadn't felt before. I quickly consented to a cystoscopy in the hospital, though I was afraid of what my doctor might find. Imagine my relief when he told me that he saw no signs of IC or anything else wrong with my bladder! Other tests however, detected some serious gynecological troubles that required a complete hysterectomy. I was sure the origin of my pain was gynecological, and a hysterectomy would take care of everything.

I was wrong. I developed a severe bladder infection while in the hospital for the hysterectomy, and was sent home on antibiotics. Several weeks later, routine urine cultures showed the infection was gone but I continued to be in daily unrelenting, bladder and urethral pain. It felt like hot acid was being poured through my body, and I had the constant urge to urinate. My lower abdomen and back ached from the moment I opened my eyes in the morning to the instant I fell asleep. Burning pain became my constant companion during the day, and prodded me out of my slumber at night. Repeated urine cultures still showed no bladder infection. Finally in 1990, a year after my hysterectomy, I had another cystoscopy. Finally, my bladder had the characteristic appearance that confirmed a diagnosis of IC. It had been six long years since the first hint of trouble. Feeling both relieved and devastated, I began the slow process of grieving for the former life I had lost, while picking up the pieces and exploring the options that my new existence presented me.

The food connection

Soon after my diagnosis in 1990, I began to suspect that something I was eating was making my bladder symptoms worse. As the year came to a close, I embarked on an elimination diet to try to pinpoint the problem food. Weeks and then months passed by, and as item after item appeared to make my pain worse and I grew more disheartened. At the end of a full year, I finally had a list of about forty different foods that I knew I had to stay away from. The worst part was, every recipe I had contained at least one of those foods. All of my family's favorites were off limits for me! I was angry and frustrated every time I was confronted with meal planning. Cooking, which used to be a joy, became an onerous task . The idea of eating at a restaurant terrified me, too. Who knows what may be in the food? I was too afraid to give it a try. For me, the events of one particular day sum up how I felt during that low point of my life.

One day I had talked myself up for the task of the weekly grocery shopping. I told myself that surely in a store with thousands of packaged, easy-to-cook items, there was something I could eat. Energy, determination, and a positive attitude had always helped me overcome obstacles in the past. I just knew it would this time too. I began my systematic search with the first aisle of the market, cheeses and deli items. I carefully scanned labels. Nothing to eat there. I went quickly through the liquor section and the soft drink section. Nothing there. I continued down each aisle in an item-by-item search, stopping to scan labels on anything that looked promising.

As I passed by whole sections of tomato products and Mexican food, rows of salad dressings and snack foods, I became more and more frustrated, then angry. Look at all these great products for everyone but me! By the time I got to the middle of the store, my shopping cart was still empty, my bladder was aching, and I was feeling alone and depressed. I felt like a child whose nose was pressed against the window of a candy store, on the outside looking in at the goodies life had to offer.

I ran out of the store, crying. I sobbed while driving home, and in my distraction ran a stop sign right in front of a police cruiser. The officer pulled me over, and looking at my tearful face, matter-of-factly asked if I noticed the stop sign. I said "no", and as I was hunting in my purse for my license, I tried to explain about IC and why I was so upset. He just gave me a cold glare. My bladder hurt worse than ever and I really had to get home to use the bathroom. I silently accepted the ticket and his gruff admonition to "pay attention more." When I got home, I flew down the hall and into the bathroom. But I was so tense and upset, I couldn't urinate a drop.

Sound familiar? You too may be able to recount similar times when frustration and physical pain just got the better of you. It's an experience that all of us with IC can relate to.

Finding support

If you've just been diagnosed, you will find the readjustment and accommodation to having a chronic illness brings with it a lot of emotions. Be easy on yourself and give yourself time to adjust. It's hard work to gain a different perspective on the world, a new set of priorities, and a new way of relating to food, to sex, to traveling, working, and recreation. It takes time to get used to the idea of daily medication, daily exercise, and constant attention to diet, as inconvenient but necessary realities.

For many of us, the anger and sense of loss we experience when we are first diagnosed, lead to a period of soul-searching and spiritual renewal. It can be a time of evaluating relationships and reinventing oneself. Thomas, a former banker, says, "I was hurting so bad I just couldn't handle the stress of my job anymore. So I quit and found a new line of work, which I actually like better. I don't think I would have done it if it hadn't been for the IC." As someone once told me, thorns can also have roses.

Though I have been fortunate to have the emotional support of family members, I'm especially glad to have found others with interstitial cystitis at an IC support group that meets near my house. These days I also meet new friends through the convenience of the computer. (The internet is a great tool for finding information and contacting others while not having to leave the comfort of home— or the proximity of a bathroom).

I'm grateful for the compassionate and supportive people I have found at my local IC group and in the electronic IC community on the internet. They've all touched my life in some way and I'm especially thankful for the time many of them took out of their lives to help me understand IC, and to give me the benefit of their experience in coping with it. I'm still learning more each day and still meeting new "IC friends".

I'll leave you with this parting thought on the subject of friends, a bit of advice which was given to me by a man who suffers from chronic debilitating migraines: "No matter how bad your condition is, you'll feel better if you stop viewing your body as a war zone and everything you do as a skirmish with the enemy. You and that body are together for the duration— for pete's sake make friends."

These days, inventing new recipes for my IC-safe diet has become just one of the things I do for my long-suffering "friend" and life-long companion, my body. I hope you and yours enjoy these recipes as much as I do.

ACKNOWLEDGMENTS

The road that led me to write this cookbook has been a long one. For several years it frustrated me that bookstores carried rows of cookbooks for people with diabetes, heart disease, and other medical conditions, but nothing at all for those of us with interstitial cystitis (IC). Then a few years ago I met Lois Arias and Barb Willis through an electronic message board on America Online. What a relief to find others who shared my frustrations and what a comfort to have such good friends!

Without Lois and Barb this project would never have gotten off the ground. The three of us knew there was a need for a cookbook, but it was Lois who lit a fire under us to actually *do* something. That winter we happily planned to write a cookbook together, linked across the country by our home computers. If it needs to be done, we thought, then let's do it ourselves!

But as one man with IC so aptly put it, "Having IC means never being able to say, 'this is for certain'." While Barb, Lois, and I were beginning the process of organizing, before any of us had the chance to write so much as a word of text, problems arose.

Lois' IC was flaring, she was physically exhausted by life's demands on her time, and her family desperately needed what energy and physical strength she could muster. The IC patient community on America Online was growing rapidly too. As "old-timers" to IC, both Lois and Barb were spending dozens of hours a week personally answering e-mail questions from distraught newly-diagnosed patients.

Stress, as we all know, tends to make our bladder problems worse. Something had to give. So Lois, being the wonderful wife, mother and person that she is, put her family's needs and those of other IC patients first, and bowed out of the cookbook-writing effort. Barb too had a crisis, as she endured a severe flare in her IC topped off by a flare in her fibromyalgia that left her immobilized, barely able to participate in the America Online group. Soon even more medical problems beset her and Barb too, regretfully gave up on our cookbook idea.

I sat down and had a long talk with my husband. Should I quit too? Though my body was temporarily in a cooperative mood, I was afraid to begin working on a book knowing the ups and downs of this disease. I felt I was facing a Mount Everest of commitment. How would I feel months or years down the road if I too had to give up due to medical problems ...after working so hard? My husband looked squarely at me and asked, "How will you feel about yourself if you never even *try*?" It was a thought-provoking question to mull over. In the end I resolved to begin again— to start afresh and begin working alone on a new book. And so, this book had its beginnings.

But as they say, closing a door on one part of your life opens a window of opportunity on another. Barb and Lois donated their time, love, and experience to the IC community on America Online. Later when Lois left to pursue other goals in her life, her role was assumed by another dedicated volunteer, known affectionately to those online as "Cath767". People like these have helped change hundreds of lives for the better. Long after there is a cure for interstitial cystitis and this book is forgotten, their personal contributions will no doubt be remembered by the people whose lives they touched. It's volunteers like these, working alone or in support groups, within organizations or on their own, who are responsible for many of the wonderful and supportive resources which have become available to IC patients over the last ten years.

Although I can't mention each and every one by name, I especially wish to thank the thousands of people with interstitial cystitis who frequent the internet message boards, attend local support group meetings, volunteer for the ICA's national telephone support network, help maintain the IC Network's enormous website, or find other ways to generously share their experience with this disease so that we all may benefit.

I give thanks to my husband, Charlie, who has endured many "experimental" dinners over the years I've had IC, and never once admonished me about playing with the food. I thank all my family for the years of taste-testing my food adventures at family get-togethers, and for their understanding and compassion through all the frustration that IC brings. I especially thank my mom, Viva, for her advice and encouragement over the many years I've had IC, and my dad, Forbes, for raising me to be the kind of tough cookie that could see this project through to completion.

Especially to fellow IC patients Jill Osborne, Barbara Hyatt, Sue Cogburn, Barb Willis, Lois Arias, Bronwyn McGowen, and Karen Thurston I owe a debt of gratitude for sharing with me their IC dietary wisdom. I want to extend a heartfelt thanks to Bruce Henderson, Angela Meiss, John Frankfort, and all the others who helped this project along in large or little ways. I'd like to commend Bob Anderson at KNI for his patience and helpful suggestions, and thank the people behind Freeman Family Trust Publications who had faith in my work. And of course, I owe a lot to my capable team of doctors, whose medical skills kept me going through the worst symptom flares, and without whom I never would have been able to complete this.

But there is one to whom I owe more than all others, and whose blessing and timely assistance made my life with chronic illness bearable and this book a reality. And so, saving the greatest debt of gratitude to last, I wish to thank God.

INTRODUCTION

Interstitial cystitis (IC) is a chronic urinary tract disease characterized by bladder, urethral, and general pelvic pain, as well as urgency and frequency of urination. Those of us with IC often require dozens of trips to the bathroom per day, and wake numerous times per night with burning pain and urinary urgency. People with IC will frequently complain that it feels like they have a bladder infection, but routine laboratory tests reveal no infection. Interstitial cystitis occurs primarily in women, and often the symptoms first appear in midlife. Young women, men, and (rarely) children can also suffer from it. The symptoms wax and wane, in irregular and unpredictable cycles of remissions and flare-ups, leaving the IC sufferer often feeling helpless and without control over his or her life. Although there is currently no cure and the cause has yet to be found, various treatments are now available to ease the symptoms.

As a longtime IC sufferer myself, I have found that patience is more than just a virtue. If you have IC, it's a necessity. The chief drawback of many of the IC treatments available is that they take time to work. With some, it may take months before one can expect any symptomatic relief. Not all treatments work for every person with IC, either. It takes time to find out which one works for you, and that often entails going through several that don't, before you find the one that does. It is a frustrating situation for all of us with IC. It's frustrating for doctors, too, in that they cannot tell in advance which patient is likely to be helped by which kind of treatment. While we wait in hopeful anticipation that research will give us some answers, there is one step that many people with IC will tell you makes an immediate and tremendous difference in their urinary pain and frequency. It is diet.

"The IC diet" as patients call it, is simply a list of foods that exacerbate bladder symptoms. The list is slightly different for each person, and again, it takes time to figure out exactly which foods cause problems for you. Given enough time and the willingness to experiment with many foods, most IC sufferers can come up with a long list of foods to avoid. In talking with others who share the affliction, they also soon find out that in many ways everyone's list of foods to avoid is similar. The Interstitial Cystitis Association (ICA), headquartered in New York, has tapped into the collective dietary experience of patients and published a handy pamphlet listing the foods that IC patients find most troublesome. (I found my trigger foods through an elimination diet similar to the one allergists recommend. You may want to do the same, but using the ICA's list as a guide and starting point will save you a lot of time. For a small fee they will send you a copy of their pamphlet. Their address is listed in Appendix C.)

For many years the idea of IC symptoms being affected by diet was controversial. Doctors would scoff at patients who said their pain and urinary frequency diminished when they avoided certain foods. But in recent years, IC research has given credibility to what patients had been saying all along. More and more doctors are seeing diet as a valuable tool in the management of IC.

Interstitial cystitis is a disease of many faces. Some people have only urinary frequency and no pain. A few people have pain and hardly any frequency, but most have both. Extreme urgency to urinate is another difficulty of many with IC. All these symptoms can be anywhere from mild to severe. The pain can be dull and aching, to sharp and stabbing. Patients often describe the sharp pain as being like knives in the bladder, electric shocks, or like hot acid. Some IC sufferers use the restroom only six or seven times per day, while others feel the urge to urinate constantly, and do so as many as fifty times per day. Just as the pain and frequency is an individual matter, so is our response to dietary factors. You may find that diet doesn't affect your symptoms very much. Or you may find that even a few nibbles of forbidden foods can put you in bed with agony that lasts days. Mary, who has had IC for several years, sums up another frustrating aspect: "Some days I can eat a little bit of cheese with no problem, and other days it just gets me— wham! It drives me crazy trying to figure out why, or what I did differently!"

I am not a doctor, so I won't go into any of the medical aspects of IC, or any treatments for the disease, in this book. That is beyond the scope of what is essentially a cookbook, and definitely beyond the scope of my education and experience. Like you, I'm just a person with IC sharing her experiences, and a few strategies that I've found to be helpful.

In all cases, I encourage open and honest communication with your doctor. Being assertive, knowledgeable, and prepared for visits to your doctor will reap many rewards, both physical and emotional. Building a solid partnership with your doctor is essential to overcoming the medical and emotional problems that a chronic illness hands us. Though we may not be able to change which way the wind blows, we can set our sails to get us going in the right direction. We can have a satisfying, rewarding, and joy-filled life while still having IC.

Most IC patients I know follow some form of the IC diet while they are also taking various prescription medications to treat their bladder symptoms. I've also met a few patients like Bronwyn, who says her IC is so well under control that she can now pretty much dispense with the dietary restrictions. Although her doctor has her on a treatment that works well for her, she did have to follow a strict diet at first, until the symptoms were under control. Some foods can interact with some medications though, and you may have other medical conditions that need to be taken into consideration, so please consult your own doctor or other health practitioner before trying anything new, including radical dietary changes.

Soon after my IC diagnosis in 1990, while following an elimination diet, I began collecting recipes containing only ingredients that I knew I could safely eat. Soon I was bored with the few recipes I had, and began to improvise and develop my own IC-safe recipes. Finding or creating recipes that use such a limited palette of ingredients and flavors is difficult. In this book, I am sharing some of my favorites.

To get the most out of the book, you should probably set aside some time to sit down and read Part One before trying the recipes. Part One is loaded with background information and numerous practical suggestions to make the experience of cooking and eating meals more fun and worry-free. Many more short essays and ideas are included throughout Part Two, the recipe section. Part Three is a treasure trove of resources for IC patients, listing where to find food items, as well as places to get more information.

To make this book as helpful and inclusive as possible, I've attempted to be very restrictive in the ingredients used in the recipes. I wanted a person with even the most severe case of IC, (and perhaps several other medical conditions) to be able to use the majority of recipes here. I didn't want to settle for another cookbook with "something for everyone." Although the limited list of ingredients was very challenging, I hope this book has "a lot for everyone." If this book makes even one person's days in the shadow of this disease more rewarding and enjoyable, I will count the writing of it worthwhile.

PART ONE

AN INTERSTITIAL CYSTITIS DIET

There are many foods that are notorious for exacerbating bladder symptoms and some of them seem to be worse than others. We often say that eating certain foods will cause "flares." A "flare" is what we call those periods when the IC symptoms worsen. Not everyone has dramatic "flares." Some who have very severe cases have symptoms so bad that they can't recognize any ups and downs. Only when appropriate medical treatment begins to affect the pain, urgency, and frequency level, do they start to notice the ups and downs of "flares." Then there are the lucky few who say that foods don't seem to affect their symptoms much. Wouldn't we all like to be that lucky?

Bottled cranberry juice cocktail, which doctors often advise for patients with bladder infections, is one of the foremost offenders for almost everyone with IC. Many years ago, when I was getting chronic bladder infections, I drank cranberry juice because my doctor said it might help fight the infection. It didn't cause any pain. Now that I have IC, it only takes a little cranberry juice to put me in bed with a heating pad. One newly-diagnosed woman was very surprised to find it was cranberry juice that was setting off her flares. She posted this on an internet IC newsgroup: "Do you mean to tell me that cranberry juice is bad for an IC bladder?!! Oh migosh... I've been drinking quarts of it! I thought it was supposed to be good for bladders... No wonder my pain is just getting worse and worse!"

Not all the foods on an IC diet are so universally problematic. There are individual differences in how people react. Food allergies and other medical conditions may also be factors in what foods each person is sensitive to. Bananas have never given me a problem, but I have heard from others who cannot tolerate them. Lori, who has had IC for four years, is able to drink reduced-acid orange juice. She was very excited when she found it in her supermarket, and urged me to try it. I did, but found it was still acid enough to cause me a two-day flare in bladder pain. That's just one of the challenges people with IC have to deal with. You have to take other people's advice and experience "with a grain of salt" as my grandmother would say.

Another challenging aspect of our relationship with food is the variable response we can have. One day I'll "cheat" and have a bit of chocolate. No problem. Yet a few weeks later, I'll do the same thing, and it causes a major flare in my bladder pain. There's also the delayed response we can sometimes have: that piece of chocolate may cause pain and urgency in minutes, or the same burning agony may not set in until the next day.

In writing this cookbook, I have excluded as many offensive foods as possible from the recipes. Some foods I have listed on the next page as Group 1. These foods don't appear in any form, in any of the recipes in this book. All of them are identified in publications by the Interstitial Cystitis Association (ICA), as triggering IC symptoms.

Although researchers may have some medical theories about why these foods cause bladder pain, I based their exclusion from my recipes on the answers to two questions: First, how many people have a problem with this food? And second, how easy is the food to avoid? Later I will discuss some of these foods in more detail.

GROUP 1 FOODS

NOT USED IN ANY RECIPE

aged cheeses (i.e., cheddar, Roquefort, brie)
aged, processed, cured, & smoked meats
  and fish (or any animal product with nitrites)
anchovies
apples
apricots
aspartame (i.e., Nutrasweet)
avocadoes
bananas
beer
berries (except blueberries and blackberries)
caffeine
cantaloupes
carbonated drinks
caviar
cherries (sour and sweet)
chicken livers
chocolate
citric acid
citrus fruit and citrus juices
coffee
corned beef
cranberries and cranberry juice
fava beans
grapes
"hot" spices (these include cayenne, chiles
  and chile powder, cloves, cumin, curry
  powder, fenugreek, & paprika)
lima beans
mayonnaise
miso
MSG (monosodium glutamate)
nectarines
peaches
pineapples
plums
pomegranates
raw globe or green onions
red wine
rhubarb
rye and sourdough bread
saccharine
salad dressing (commercially
  prepared)
sodium benzoate or
  potassium benzoate
soy sauce (except some
  low-sodium)
strawberries
tea
tofu
tomatoes
vinegar
white wine and other
  alcoholic beverages
  when not cooked
yogurt

There are a few foods *not* listed above which can also be problematic for people with IC. For the sake of simplicity, I've called these foods Group 2. Rather than exclude them totally, for various reasons I've limited their use to a small percentage of the recipes. For those with very sensitive bladders, I've also provided some safer alternatives to these limited-use foods when they appear in recipes.

GROUP 2 FOODS
VERY LIMITED USE IN REC!PES

◆ **Cooking sherry.** This is the only alcoholic beverage used in any recipe, and it is only used in a very few cases where the alcohol boils off. (See Wine and Beer, page 42, for more information). In my personal experience, many sweet white dessert wines (such as cream sherry) work well for flavoring foods in situations where the alcohol evaporates.

◆ **Cooked globe onions, cooked green onions. Raw chives in very small amounts.** When cooked, onions are less of a problem for many people. (See Onions, page 54).

◆ **Low-sodium soy sauce.** Some people report that although regular soy sauce bothers their bladder, they can use certain brands of soy sauce which are labelled "low-sodium." (See Monosodium Glutamate, page 51, and products list in Appendix B).

◆ **Nuts (other than almonds, pine nuts, and cashews).** Nuts are almost never the main ingredient of a recipe. When we eat them it tends to be in small amounts. Some people say they can have nuts of any kind without a problem. For those who can indulge, I've offered a couple of wonderful recipes that are best made with peanuts or pecans. (Though almonds, cashews, and pine nuts are usually safe, watch out for preservatives and other irritating or allergenic additives).

◆ **Preservatives and artificial ingredients.** There are thousands of these ingredients in our food, and the vast majority don't bother most people. But many of us who have IC do react to certain artificial ingredients. Unfortunately, the reactions can be individual and unpredictable. Artificial ingredients are eliminated from almost all of the recipes here, but a few of them do have certain products (like chicken broth) where one is likely to encounter additives. In such cases, a distinctive symbol is placed next to the recipe ingredient and a list is provided (in Appendix B) of alternative natural, or artificial ingredient-free products. (See Part Two, Key to Recipe Symbols).

◆ **Ripe blackberries.** Some people with IC seem to be able to eat small amounts of this berry if they are very ripe. Again, there are only a couple of recipes with this ingredient, and they are instances where the acidity of the berry is moderated by another very alkaline ingredient. (There are many berries that haven't been widely evaluated by IC patients. Some are only popular in a certain part of the country. Boysenberries and olallieberries fall into that category. Use your own judgement with these).

Besides just avoiding certain foods, there are a number of other interesting food "phenomena" that people with IC report. Here are a few worth mentioning.

Bananas: If bananas bother your bladder, but you want to indulge in eating them now and then, you may be better off eating ones that are slightly green. (Bananas that are very ripe have been reported to be high in tyramine.)

Chocolate: Chocolate has a lot of caffeine, among other things. If you just can't resist the dark, sweet temptation of chocolate, you may have less problems with milk chocolate than with dark chocolate. As for candy, a thin coating or a few chocolate chips are better than a solid bar, too. It may be a personal quirk, but I seem to have better luck "cheating" with chocolate early in the day, rather than late in the evening.

Dried cranberries: A few people have reported that they can actually tolerate dried cranberries while other cranberry products cause them intense pain. Again, this may be a personal quirk, so try these at your own risk.

Raisins: Some people who wouldn't think of eating grapes, can eat raisins.

Tea: Although most tea and tea-containing products are "out" due to their bladder-provoking caffeine, some herb teas are okay. But watch out for those listing rose hips as a major ingredient (they often have a high ascorbic acid content).

Yogurt: For some unknown reason, a few people with IC have said that they can eat frozen yogurt, while refrigerated yogurt is off limits for them. What's the difference? I wish I knew. I'm one of the fortunate ones who can eat a bit of frozen yogurt now and then as long as its not right before bed.

One last note on the subject of food quirks. You may find medications affect the way you respond to foods, too. Before I began taking the prescription drug Elmiron, I could safely eat a ripe plum now and then. But no way would I think of trying something as spicy hot as Kung Pao Chicken. After nine months of taking Elmiron though, I found I could once again have the Kung Pao Chicken— yet the plums I once tolerated, had become real bladder-burners!

COEXISTING MEDICAL CONDITIONS AND DIET

Some IC sufferers appear to be in perfect health except for their bladder problems. But epidemiological studies have shown that unfortunately, this isn't the case for all of us. No one knows why, but significant numbers of IC patients have certain other diseases or syndromes along with the IC. (A "syndrome" is just a collection of signs and symptoms that tend to occur together). These coexisting conditions can make coping with the IC more difficult.

Many of us have joint or muscle pains, and have been diagnosed with arthritis or fibromyalgia syndrome (FMS). Others have been diagnosed with something doctors call irritable bowel syndrome (IBS). For some women with IC, vulvar pain (vulvodynia) accompanies the bladder pain, urgency, and urinary frequency. IC patients frequently have migraines, sinus trouble, or asthma, and a lot of us have allergies to what we breathe, to what we eat, or to medications. Recent research has revealed that large numbers of us have sensitive skin.

For many years, IC was thought of as a "hysterical" or psychological disorder of women. Then, beginning in the 1980's, and largely thanks to the efforts of the Interstitial Cystitis Association, the medical community began to accept IC as a urological disease. Today, research on IC is expanding and evidence has been found which indicates that in some people at least, IC may be a localized effect of a more systemic disorder. The attention of the medical community is now being focused as well on some of the other physical complaints common to IC patients. Doctors are hoping that by identifying and studying the links between IC and some of these other diseases and physical complaints, they can shed some light on the cause of IC.

Doctors and patients have found that, like IC itself, some IC-associated conditions respond to dietary changes. Though the recipes in this book are aimed primarily at avoiding symptoms of interstitial cystitis (bladder pain, urinary urgency, and frequency) I have tried to keep in mind the needs of those who have more than one medical problem. Many recipes are easily adaptable. The following pages contain some information on diet as it relates to food allergy, irritable bowel syndrome, fibromyalgia, vulvodynia, migraines, and candida albicans (yeast) infections. Juggling the requirements of several differing diets can be challenging. To help those who need a vegetarian diet or who have vulvodynia, I've also included two special indexes in Appendix E. But please— first and foremost— talk with your doctor about any dietary changes you are thinking of making. It is especially important to have professional guidance if you are excluding several food groups, or large numbers of foods from your diet.

If you have religious or cultural dietary requirements, have complex medical needs, want to lose weight, or would just like to be sure you are getting proper nutrition— you may benefit by talking to a nutrition professional, such as a registered dietician. A dietician can help you plan a diet that provides for your body's needs and also fits your lifestyle and pocketbook. Your doctor may be able to recommend one. Hospitals are excellent sources of referrals. The American Dietetic Association or your state's Dietetic Association also gives referrals. Information on contacting the American Dietetic Association appears at the back of the book, in Appendix C.

Food Allergies and Intolerances

If you try sticking to an IC diet and still feel that foods may be contributing to your bladder symptoms, you may want to investigate whether or not you have food allergies or intolerances. In a survey of IC patients done at Scripps Institute, 25 % reported having food allergies. Another study published in 1997 found that around 42% of the IC patients surveyed had been diagnosed with allergies by a physician. In that study, allergies were found to be the most common disorder associated with IC, and may be almost twice as prevalent among IC patients, as in the general population.

From a doctor's perspective, food allergies and food intolerances are different. According to the American Academy of Allergy, Asthma and Immunology (AAAAI), food allergy involves an abnormal reaction by the immune system, whereas a food intolerance is an abnormal physical reaction that does not appear to be caused by the immune system. If you have a true food allergy, you are reacting to a food which contains an allergen. The allergen is that part of the food which provokes the body's response, and it is usually a protein. (Vegetables as wells as meat, contain proteins). Even after they are cooked or have undergone digestion in the intestines, most allergens can still cause problems for an allergic individual .

Some common foods that provoke allergic symptoms in many people are wheat, dairy, peanuts, eggs, soy, and shellfish. Many more foods may provoke symptoms in certain people.

Some food groups exhibit "cross-reactivity." That is, if you are allergic to one food in that food group, you may become allergic to others as well. Peanuts, for instance, are members of the same family (legumes) as peas, lima beans and soy beans. If you have an allergy to peanuts, you may develop one to lima beans. You would be less likely to develop one to almonds, say, because they are members of another food family.

You may only be allergic to certain parts of a food: people with an egg allergy usually react only to the white of the egg. If the food is a fruit, ripening may affect how you respond to the food also. Tomatoes are notorious for becoming more allergenic as they ripen.

A food intolerance is usually caused by some factor in the food other than a protein. Lactose intolerance is a physical reaction caused by the body's inability to digest a kind of sugar that is in milk. Food intolerance reactions can be caused by substances which naturally occur in the food, or they may be triggered by additives. The following additives are some of those commonly thought to cause adverse reactions: benzoates,

BHT and BHA, FD&C dyes (especially yellow #5), MSG, nitrates and nitrites, and sulfites.

An allergist can help you determine if you have any true food allergies. Regardless of whether you have allergies or intolerances, he or she may recommend an "elimination diet" to help pinpoint the problem foods. This kind of diet entails temporarily eliminating every possible problem food from one's diet, then gradually adding back the foods one at a time, while watching for the return of symptoms. Once you have determined which foods cause problems, your doctor may recommend a treatment plan.

To a patient who may be experiencing everything from skin rashes to abdominal cramps or difficulty breathing, the clinical difference between an intolerance and an allergy is of little importance— we just want relief. And often that can only be obtained through complete avoidance of the offending foods. If you, or others in your family have multiple food allergies/intolerances as well as interstitial cystitis, cooking can be especially difficult. A good book you might want to have in your kitchen is *The Allergy Self-help Cookbook,* by Marjorie Hurt-Jones, R.N. (Rodale Press). It has many recipes which are free from wheat, eggs, milk, corn, yeast, and sugar. Some are IC-safe, and some can be made IC-safe with a few changes.

The AAAAI puts out several helpful items, including a very informative eight-page booklet for patients, on the subject of food intolerances and food allergies. (For the address and phone of the American Academy of Allergy, Asthma and Immunology, see Appendix C).

Irritable Bowel Syndrome (IBS)

Irritable bowel syndrome has been estimated to affect 10-15% of the population in the United States, with perhaps 3% of the population having a severe enough case to consult a physician for the condition. In contrast, recent estimates show symptoms of irritable bowel syndrome (IBS) may occur in 20-34% of all IC patients. According to a study of IC-associated conditions published in the medical journal *Urology*, irritable bowel syndrome was the second most common IC-associated disease. In that study, more than 33% of the over 2400 IC patients surveyed, reported symptoms of IBS. The same study indicated that about 27% of IC patients had their IBS diagnosed by a physician. This ground-breaking study also noted that irritable bowel syndrome tended to precede the symptoms of IC for those patients who had both.

According to the U.C.L.A. Neuroenteric Disease Section and the International Foundation for Functional Gastrointestinal Disorders (IFFGD), the abdominal pain characteristic of IBS is triggered by spasms of the smooth muscles which form the lower gastrointestinal tract, or colon. The nerves that control these colon muscles are unusually active, so diarrhea, constipation, or alternating bouts of each, are common symptoms. The pain of IBS is thought to be a result of nerve endings in the colon that are unusually sensitive to any stimuli. Although the cause of this colonic disturbance is not completely understood, doctors can perform tests to diagnose it and give patients various medications to help alleviate the symptoms. (I was pleasantly surprised to find that an antispasmodic medication I use for my IBS symptoms, also helps my IC bladder spasms).

Some people with IBS find that certain foods exacerbate their symptoms. The IFFGD advocates maintaining a food-and-symptoms diary for a minimum of one week to help identify your IBS food triggers. If you have multiple food intolerances, it may take longer to find them all.

The list of offending foods will vary from person to person, but certain foods are notorious triggers. Corn, wheat, sorbitol (an artificial sweetener found in many products including toothpaste), and monosodium glutamate (MSG), are common offenders. For some with IBS, excessive dietary fats, such as are found in hamburger for instance, can be a trigger. (And although it is illegal, some supermarkets grind up their leftover pork trimmings with their ground beef. If you have a sensitivity to pork, this may be another reason hamburger affects your IBS). IC patients with irritable bowel syndrome often say that aged cheeses, red wine, and aspartame (an artificial sweetener) can cause bowel symptoms as well as bladder symptoms for them. Guar gum is another substance that can cause bowel trouble.

If, in addition to having IC, you are one of the 17% of Americans who are unable to digest milk products, you may find that abdominal cramping is triggered by the milk sugar, lactose. An enzyme called lactase (available over-the-counter in drugstores and supermarkets), can ease abdominal symptoms for people who are lactose intolerant. If that fails to help, you may find relief by avoiding all dairy products (except butter).

Any food which causes excessive gas in the lower gastrointestinal tract can also provoke the painful spasms of IBS. If gas causes problems for you, try avoiding the cruciferous vegetables such as broccoli, brussels sprouts, cauliflower, cabbage and kale. You may also want to watch out for soups and stews made with dried beans and dried peas. Much of the "gas" difficulty with dried beans and peas can be avoided by making your own soups and stews and being sure that the beans soak overnight before cooking. Soaking overnight causes a chemical reaction to take place inside the bean which reduces the amount of an indigestible sugar responsible for forming gas in the intestines.

I spoke with one young mother taking pentosan polysulfate (Elmiron) for her IC. She said the drug caused her increased intestinal gas, which would trigger the abdominal cramps of her IBS. A vegetarian, she found that eating gas-producing vegetables only made matters worse. In desperation she tried Beano, an over-the-counter product sold in drugstores. It seemed to help with the gas, she said, even when she wasn't eating the gas-producing vegetables. I too have found Beano to be very useful for combatting food-produced gas and the accompanying IBS symptoms.

Doctors often advise IBS patients to increase the natural fiber in their diet. According to an IFFGD 1995 Symposium Report, increased fiber will help relieve constipation in IBS patients only if they also increase the amount of fluids they consume. (Unfortunately for those with IC, drinking more fluids may mean more trips to the bathroom). It was also found that while fiber helps some people, others will experience increased bloating and pain. For those people, a diet quite low in fiber may be beneficial.

The "bland diet" is one that many doctors recommend for people with stomach and intestinal disorders. It is a diet low in natural fiber. Barbara, a cheerful lady in her fifties who has had IC for several years, also battled bouts of IBS diarrhea until a nurse told her to try the bland diet. "Boy, it's been the only thing that works for me!", she says. On a bland diet one usually avoids citrus and tomatoes, beans, coarse whole-grained cereals and breads, raw fruit and vegetables, smoked meats, vegetables in the cabbage family, cheeses, and caffeine. Spices that one should avoid on a bland diet include: cayenne, chili powder, cloves, horseradish, mustard (dry), peppercorns, red pepper (red, ground or crushed), and black pepper. (Many of these items are ones that IC patients watch out for anyway.)

One home remedy that some people say actually helps their symptoms of IBS, is peppermint oil. Several IBS sufferers who post on internet newsgroups have reported favorable results with enteric-coated peppermint oil capsules. But a word of warning: According to author Devin Starlanyl, M.D. (*Fibromyalgia & Chronic Myofascial Pain Syndrome*, New Harbinger Publications, 1996), the enteric coating is there to keep it from breaking down in the stomach and causing gas. Any gas of course, can make IBS worse. Dr. Starlanyl advises her patients with IBS to only try peppermint oil if it is in enteric-coated capsules. Plain peppermint oil is strong, irritating to the gastrointestinal tract, and may make you feel worse. Enteric-coated peppermint oil capsules are carried by some of the sources listed in Appendix B.

For more information on IBS, and organizations who can help those with IBS, see the resource list in Appendix C. You may also find one of the books on the subject quite interesting. (See the Reading List in Appendix D.)

Fibromyalgia Syndrome (FMS)

Fibromyalgia (sometimes called "fibromyalgia syndrome" or FMS) is a cluster of symptoms, the most prominent of which are generalized muscular pain and fatigue. Although fibromyalgia may feel like joint pain, it actually affects the muscles. Unlike arthritis, it doesn't cause deformities of the joints. Doctors disagree on the exact numbers, but somewhere between 10% and 60% of IC patients report symptoms consistent with fibromyalgia. One recent nationwide survey of hundreds of IC patients found that approximately 17% had been formally diagnosed with fibromyalgia. The survey also found that the onset of fibromyalgia usually occurred after the onset of IC symptoms.

About 90% of people with fibromyalgia describe fatigue, lack of energy, difficulty in concentrating, or lack of sleep as things that bother them. Their body seems "stiff" and hard to move after remaining in one position for very long. Migraine headaches and symptoms of irritable bowel syndrome (IBS) are common in fibromyalgia too. According to Daniel Clauw M.D., in an article appearing in *American Family Physician*, 75% of fibromyalgia patients exhibit evidence of mitral valve prolapse and 84% complain of numbness or tingling in the extremities. Dr. Clauw also notes that many display a wide array of apparently "allergic" symptoms including chronic rhinitis and nasal congestion. (While writing this book I came across an article in a medical journal linking fibromyalgia and symptoms of sinus irritation. I knew I had the muscular pain of fibromyalgia, but until that moment it never occurred to me to connect the runny nose I get every time I eat dinner, with my fibromyalgia.)

Sleep disturbances are associated with this disorder, and lack of deep sleep tends to correlate with the muscular symptom flares. Foods that tend to cause heartburn for you, or create gas that keeps you awake, should definitely be avoided. Neurologist Dr. David Nye suggests his fibromyalgia patients avoid the following because the caffeine or alcohol in them tend to interfere with the deep, restorative sleep that fibromyalgia sufferers need: coffee, chocolate, soft drinks containing caffeine, beer, wine, and other alcoholic beverages. (Be sure to read beverage labels. It's not just cola drinks that contain caffeine. Even clear sodas such as Mountain Dew can have significant amounts of caffeine).

Many IC patients with fibromyalgia report cravings for sweets and other carbohydrate-dense foods. Dr. Devin Starlanyl, a physician and fellow fibromyalgia sufferer, describes a condition called reactive hypoglycemia which can cause sugar craving. Reactive hypoglycemia is common in fibromyalgia and according to Dr. Starlanyl, may make itself known by weakness or tremors that frequently occur before meals, but are halted by eating— especially by eating sweets. When people with reactive hypoglycemia eat sugar, their body overreacts. The insulin level shoots up, then nosedives, sending the person into a drowsy stupor. Dr. Starlanyl finds that many of her fibromyalgia patients who exhibit reactive hypoglycemia also have way more yeasts in their system than average, and she feels the increased yeast burden may amplify their sugar cravings. For more information on fibromyalgia, see the list of organizations in Appendix C, and the reading list in Appendix D.

Migraines

More than a simple headache, migraines are often very intense, sometimes accompanied by nausea or visual disturbances, and usually occur on one side of the head only. The cause is unknown. One currently favored view among doctors is that migraines are triggered by blood vessels in the head which constrict and then suddenly dilate, stretching the nerves and bringing on a headache.

In the general population, there are both men and women who suffer from migraines, though women outnumber men by a wide margin. In one recent nationwide survey of IC patients, migraines were found to occur in 18% of the women and 6% of the men with IC. It is estimated that about 18% of the general population has migraines, so the prevalence of migraines in IC is not unusually high. It also appears that, from the limited research done so far, the onset of migraines precedes the onset of IC symptoms in patients who have both.

Serotonin has been investigated for its possible role in many IC-associated conditions, including migraines, fibromyalgia, and irritable bowel syndrome. It is interesting to note that some recent medical research has also focused attention on the role of the neurotransmitter, serotonin, in interstitial cystitis.

Women with both IC and migraines find that these debilitating headaches frequently occur at the beginning of their menstrual period, or that they are brought on by taking estrogen pills. My husband, who has occasional migraines, says that for him, not getting a good night's sleep can trigger one the next day.

For some migraine sufferers, food brings on headaches. According to neurologist Dr. Joel Saper, 25% of migraine sufferers can associate their headaches with a particular food. Many of the foods that trigger migraines are the same ones that cause bladder pain for IC patients. Below are some foods that many migraine sufferers say are triggers. (The * denotes foods which are excluded from all recipes in this book).

aged cheeses*
avocadoes*
bananas*
beer*
buttermilk*
caffeine in coffee and sodas*
citrus fruits and juices*
chocolate and cocoa*
freshly baked bread
lima beans*
liver, kidney and organ meat*
meats with nitrates or nitrites* (i.e., hot dogs)
MSG (monosodium glutamate)*
nuts (especially peanuts)
onions
papayas*
pea pods*
pinto beans*
raisins
sauerkraut*
sesame seeds
sunflower seeds
smoked or processed meats* (i.e., ham and bacon)
sour cream*
vinegar*
wine and alcoholic beverages (in this book, only used where the alcohol boils off)
yeast and yeast extract (autolyzed yeast)
yogurt*

For many years, doctors have recognized that some people with migraines also suffer from something called "abdominal migraines." These acute attacks of abdominal pain are sometimes accompanied by other signs and symptoms associated with migraine headaches, such as visual disturbances.

An interesting new line of investigation has been opened by Dr. Antonio Gasbarrini of Rome's Catholic University Hospital. At the 8th Congress of the International Headache Society, Dr. Gasbarrini announced that he and his colleagues have found, in a controlled study of 262 migraine headache patients, that an improvement or cure can been achieved by treating for the bacterium, Helicobacter pylori. Only the future will tell whether Dr. Gasbarrini's approach will have any practical application for IC patients who have migraines, but here is my personal experience:

I was having a terrible flare of my irritable bowel syndrome one summer and suffering from excruciating abdominal cramping and bloating. I asked my family doctor to do a test for Helicobacter pylori, the bacteria associated with stomach ulcers and stomach cancer. He was skeptical, but did it anyway. The test showed that I did indeed have some antibodies to the bacteria, but not enough to clearly indicate an infection. (I figured that since my husband had a bout of stomach problems a few years back, perhaps I had been exposed to the bacteria through him). About a year later, my husband needed to see our doctor about a prescription refill for his migraine treatment. So while he was at the doctor's office, my husband casually reminded the doctor of his past stomach problems and the results of my Helicobacter test. The doctor ordered a Helicobacter test for my husband, which turned out to be positive for an infection. After three weeks of antibiotic treatment for the stomach bacteria, much to the doctor's surprise, my husband's migraines lessened in frequency and severity.

There are several prescription medications available for migraines, and your doctor can help you find the best one for you. For more information on migraines and their treatment, there are a number of good books on the market. Some are on the technical side, while others are geared more for patients. There is also a national organization that has a wide variety of resources available to help migraine sufferers. (See Appendices C and D).

Yeast Infections

Candida albicans, or "yeast" as it is commonly called, is a fungal parasite that lives in everyone's gastrointestinal tract. It helps regulate the population of bacteria, and it is in turn kept in check by other bacteria. Candida albicans is a natural part of the gut ecology, but can get out of hand when one takes antibiotics. IC patients sometimes are given antibiotics for bladder infections or other reasons, and they also complain of a variety of symptoms some doctors think may be candida-related.

People with IC are sometimes afflicted with of a variety of fungal infections, and often they compare notes at support group meetings. For women, the fungal infections can take the form of a vaginal overgrowth of the "yeast", candida albicans. Urologist and author Dr. Kristene Whitmore writes in the ICA's publication, *Update*, that her women IC patients often have chronic, recurrent vaginal yeast infections. It has been my own experience, and that of other women IC patients I have talked to, that fungal infections in areas close to the bladder do tend to exacerbate IC bladder pain.

Like some other IC sufferers, I also seem to get fungal toenail infections very easily. My doctor tells me that the organism which causes toenail fungus is not the same as the one responsible for vaginal yeast infections, but regardless of the organism responsible, it's an annoyance in warm, humid weather, and one that I'd be happy to do without.

In the early 1980's Dr. William Crook wrote *The Yeast Connection* (Random House, 1983), which went on to become a huge success because it addressed an issue long ignored by mainstream medicine, chronic candidiasis. He described many symptoms which could be caused by a yeast overgrowth, including abdominal gas and cramping, memory problems, chronic fatigue, muscle aches, and a generally "sick all over" feeling. Crook, and other doctors since then, have found patients in whom chronic yeast infestations seemed to exacerbate health problems as diverse as fibromyalgia, vulvodynia, irritable bowel syndrome, chronic fatigue syndrome, asthma, and others.

Indiana urologist Dr. Philip Mosbaugh, in the Winter 1996 ICA (Interstitial Cystitis Assn.) *Update* , related the experience of two of his IC patients who both improved on an anti-yeast diet. As of this writing, he is undertaking a pilot study of the possible role of yeast infestations in IC.

Today, there are many books on the market about candida-related medical conditions, and most suggest a diet low in sugar and simple carbohydrates to help discourage the growth of the fungus. Most books say the diet has to be followed for quite awhile to be effective, and they warn that the symptoms may get worse for a few days at first as the yeast dies off and releases irritating substances.

Some foods allowed on these diets are pain triggers for IC bladders. Although a few IC patients say they have been helped by adhering to an anti-yeast diet, before embarking on any such diet, be sure to talk to your doctor.

Some of the foods these authors say to avoid are thought to stimulate sugar levels which encourage candida albicans, and other forbidden foods contain live or dead non-candida fungus organisms. Some authors have theorized that if your body reacts to the candida, it might also react to other forms of fungus by a mechanism doctors call "cross-reaction". Some authors also warn people not to try to treat a fungal problem without the use of antifungal medications. It is also the consensus among some who have tried anti-yeast diets, that the candida symptoms can be controlled, but a permanent cure is elusive.

First consult your doctor if you feel you may have a problem with yeast, before undertaking any drastic dietary changes. Some doctors may want to perform a candida antibody test before treating you. This is a simple blood test which will reveal if your body is producing antibodies to yeast, an indication that a yeast infestation may be responsible for your symptoms. There are serious illnesses that can cause candida-like symptoms too. Your doctor will want to rule those out. Another word of caution: on the internet message boards, there are posts by people trying very restrictive anti-yeast diets for extended periods. These people often report dramatic weight loss, possibly due to malnutrition.

Vulvodynia

Vulvodynia (sometimes referred to as "vulvar pain", "vulvovaginitis", or "pudendal neuralgia") is a disorder characterized by chronic pain in the area of the female genitalia. Burning sensations are the most common, but vulvodynia pain is very individual. The pain may be mild or intense, constant or intermittent. It is often marked by small red patches of tissue in the vaginal vestibule that are painful when touched. Before diagnosis, some women mistakenly assume they have a vaginal yeast infection. Vulvar vestibulitis, a form of vulvodynia, refers to pain caused by pressure applied to the area around the vaginal entrance.

In one study published in the journal *Urology*, around 25% of approximately 2400 IC patients reported symptoms compatible with vulvodynia, and 10.9% of the IC patients had their vulvodynia diagnosed by a physician. Because doctors feel that vulvodynia may be an under-reported disease and also because there is considerable symptom overlap between IC and vulvodynia, it is uncertain exactly how many women with interstitial cystitis may also have vulvodynia. Judging from the numbers of women I've met at various IC-related functions, it is certainly a significant number.

Although there is currently no cure for this disorder, there are a number of medications and treatment strategies that can be quite successful. Diet modification is one option that doctors may recommend to their patients with vulvodynia. Dr. Clive Solomons, a ground-breaking researcher on vulvodynia and oxalates, finds that eliminating high-oxalate foods from the diet may help many women. Response to this diet is very individualized. Diet helps some women more than others, and a food that causes symptom flares in one, may not affect another. To complicate matters further, conditions under which the food was grown may affect the oxalate level. Spinach say, from one area of the country, may have more oxalates than spinach grown in another area.

Some research findings concerning oxalate have been conflicting, yet IC patients with vulvodynia report reactions to many high-oxalate foods. Although a complete listing is beyond the scope of this book, the list on the following page contains many of the most common offenders. (The three worst, as reported by the vulvodynia sufferers I've talked to, are: spinach, rhubarb, and chocolate). Some foods not on this list may still cause vulvar pain for some women. Like the IC diet, you have to discover the individual variations for yourself. Some vulvodynia patients report that simply avoiding certain foods controls their vulvar pain. For others, diet is not sufficient to obtain relief.

The following list includes most of the foods that women with vulvodynia find troublesome, but it is far from exhaustive. Dr. Clive Solomons and the Vulvar Pain Foundation (see Appendix C) have found other foods that have somewhat lower levels of oxalates, but which still may cause problems for some women. For more specific dietary guidelines, or information on medical treatments for vulvodynia, consult your doctor and/or one of the organizations listed in Appendix C, at the back of this book.

Some Foods That Women with Vulvodynia Often Avoid:
(The * symbol denotes foods which are not found in recipes in this book).

- beets*
- beer*
- beans of all kinds (only limas* and favas* should be avoided on the IC diet)
- Blackberries, blueberries, dewberries*, gooseberries*, raspberries, strawberries*
- black pepper (except in small amounts)
- broccoli
- celery
- chard*
- citrus peel
- chocolate and cocoa*
- coffee*
- collards*
- Concord grapes*
- dandelion greens*
- dried figs*
- eggplant
- escarole*
- garbanzo beans*
- green beans
- green bell peppers (in large amounts)
- grits* and hominy*
- kale*
- kamut*
- kiwi*
- leeks*
- mustard greens*
- okra*
- parsley
- parsnips*
- pecans and peanuts
- red currants, fresh*
- rhubarb*
- rutabaga*
- sardines*
- sesame seeds
- spelt*
- spinach*
- summer squash, yellow
- sweet potatoes
- swiss chard*
- sour cherries*
- tangerines*
- tomato soups* and tomato sauces*
- tea*
- tofu*
- turnip greens*
- watercress*
- wheat germ, wheat bran & whole wheat products (includes Graham crackers)
- yams

Many women IC patients who do not have vulvodynia, nonetheless say that minor irritations of the vagina and vulvar area can trigger bladder and urethral pain. So most of us take care to avoid situations that may cause irritation (for example, excessive pool chlorine, tight spandex clothing, or spermicidal jellies.) Once we treat or eliminate the source of the vulvar irritation, we find our bladder and urethral pain subsides. But for women with both IC and vulvodynia the "vaginal-bladder connection" is even more apparent. Whenever a food triggers an intense flare of the vulvodynia, they find a flare in bladder pain and/or urethral burning often follows or accompanies it.

Susan, an energetic 30-year-old who endures the miseries of both afflictions, notes that even the smallest bit of black pepper on her food will cause a week-long flare of severe burning pain in both her urethral and vulvar area. For her and others who suffer the double whammy of vulvodynia and IC, it is hard to separate one miserable condition from the other. Sometimes it just seems to hurt everywhere "down there."

Remember that just because vaginal irritation makes your bladder hurt, doesn't mean you have vulvodynia or should follow a low-oxalate diet. But if high-oxalate foods such as spinach, green beans and parsley (which are usually not a problem for IC patients without vulvodynia) seem to irritate your bladder or urethra, you may want to see a gynecologist (or urogynecologist) familiar with the diagnosis and treatment of vulvodynia.

The importance of record-keeping

No matter how good your memory is, you will encounter times when you can't remember whether or not some food hurt your bladder last time you ate it. *Keep a written list.* What is more, physicians, disability attorneys, and insurance companies all respond well to carefully-kept records of symptoms (rated on a 1 to 10 scale of severity with notes on daily activities). Written records will help *you* figure things out too. So how nuts do you have to go with this? Not very— but let your situation and your desire to improve be your guide. The more IC-associated afflictions you have to manage, the more valuable you will find written records.

Knowing that often, as pain improves so does bladder capacity, here's what Mary's doctor asked her to do: Over the course of 48 hours, measure the urine each time you go and write down the amount. Add the amounts, then divide the total amount of urine by the total number of times you urinated in 48 hours, to get the "average voided volume." Write this figure in a diary, and repeat the procedure monthly. As he told her, doing this every so often and tracking the "average void" allows both patient and doctor to see progress (in terms of bladder capacity) over a long period, despite the daily waxing and waning of symptoms.

DIET AND GENERAL HEALTH

As a person with a chronic illness, you will no doubt find yourself constantly bombarded with advice on health and diet. You hear it from well-meaning friends and relatives. You hear it on the television, and read it in magazines. All the admonitions about what to eat seem conflicting and confusing. Eat this to avoid heart disease, eat that to avoid bone loss, eat these other things to avoid cancer. You take in all the advice and sift out the sensible from the wacky, but you are still left with the impression that there's an awful lot of do's and don'ts.

The Dietary Guidelines for Americans are seven basic principles for a healthier diet. These guidelines are the basis for all Federal nutrition information and nutrition education programs, and were developed by the U.S. Department of Agriculture and the U.S. Department of Health and Human Services. This is what they currently recommend for most average Americans, to stay healthy:

- Eat a variety of foods
- Maintain desirable weight
- Avoid too much fat, saturated fat, and cholesterol
- Eat foods with adequate starch and fiber
- Avoid too much sugar
- Avoid too much sodium
- If you drink alcoholic beverages, do so in moderation

Although the USDA's dietary guidelines seem sensible enough, you may wonder how you can possibly juggle a diet for good general health, while also avoiding so many foods which may cause urinary pain and frequency. I won't tell you it's easy. With some creativity and thought however, IC patients can stay within the IC diet and still follow sensible guidelines for healthy eating. The biggest difficulty will be boredom. And the best antidote for that is to simply have on hand a *lot* of IC-safe recipes so that you aren't faced with the same meals too often.

A word about maintaining "desirable weight": if you are taking certain medications for your IC (or other IC-associated disorders), you may put on some extra weight in spite of healthy eating habits and an exercise program. I weighed 110 pounds, give or take five pounds, ever since I was sixteen. (That's about thirty years, with time-outs for two pregnancies). At five-foot-four-inches I was slightly on the thin side, and if I exercised at all I would lose weight. Keeping my weight up was a struggle sometimes. That all changed when I began taking the muscle relaxant, cyclobenzaprine, for my fibromyalgia. For the first time in my life I was gaining unwanted pounds, and struggling to keep in a "normal" weight range for my height. Within a month I had gone from eating ice cream to offset the effect of exercise, to exercising to offset the effect of eating ice cream. I exercise regularly, and I'm not terribly overweight now, but the days of being toothpick-thin are definitely over for me. I try to think of my new fat pads as a badge of courage, an outward sign of my determination to have a life in spite of my medical problems. (I also remind myself that I don't need to live up to standards of youth and beauty promoted by advertisers who don't have to cope with what those of us with IC do).

In the course of exercising to try to offset the weight gain, I've discovered that a moderate amount of aerobic exercise is also good for my IC, IBS, and fibromyalgia symptoms. So I've been able to back off a bit on the medication, which has further helped with the weight gain. I still have to watch the sugar and fat intake more than I used to, though. I now have an appreciation of the struggles of people who need to lose weight, so many of the recipes here are relatively low-calorie and low-fat. If you enjoy baked goods, but need to reduce the fat or sugar in your diet, be sure to take a look at the section on low-fat and low-calorie baking in Appendix B.

Many people are afraid that if they follow an IC diet, they will not be getting proper nutrition, and there are several ways people deal with this fear. One typical reaction is the "shotgun" approach: take a lot of vitamin and mineral supplements in the hope that they will somehow take care of any nutritional deficits. That's an approach fraught with problems, because many vitamin and mineral preparations contain fillers that IC bladders may be sensitive to. Some forms of certain vitamins can cause an increase in bladder pain. Minerals such as iron or large amounts of calciumcarbonate can cause constipation. And although magnesium preparations are thought of as laxatives, some IC patients with IBS have had very severe bouts of constipation from magnesium supplements. See Appendix A for more on the subject of dietary supplements.

If you have a computer, a second (and saner) approach, is to buy a cookbook and dietary analysis program such as Mastercook, which can tell you the nutritional content of your meals. It won't give you an exhaustive analysis, but it will give you a general picture of your intake of important vitamins and minerals. It will also let you know how you stand in terms of cholesterol, calories, and saturated fat. In evaluating your meals, be sure to take a look at the list of nutrients in Appendix A. Each nutrient needed by the human body is available from foods that don't cause bladder pain for most IC patients.

Another good approach is to consult a dietician. This may seem to be a bit expensive, but the personal interaction and ability to ask questions of an expert may be well worth the expense if you are really worried about your diet's effect on your health. Appendix C in the back of this book lists the address of the American Dietetic Association, which can give you referrals to a registered dietician in your area. Above all don't forget to consult your doctor about any drastic dietary changes you are thinking of making. He may be able to recommend a good dietician, too.

EASING THE PHYSICAL BURDEN OF SHOPPING AND COOKING

With the increasing cost of good health care these days, no one has money to waste, especially people suffering from debilitating conditions like IC. We want bargains and good value for our money. But because we frequently don't feel well, it can be difficult to shop for food or stand on one's feet for hours cooking complicated meals. Even though I love to cook, I still find cooking a burden when I'm in severe pain. Here are some time- and money-saving strategies that other IC patients have found helpful.

Shopping strategies

◆ **Buy food in large quantities.** Shopping at warehouse-type outlets can save money if you have the room to store food properly. Large quantity purchases generally cost less per unit, but they are good buys only if you can use them up before they spoil. I try to buy things that store well for long periods such as paper goods, oatmeal, and canned goods.

◆ **Make fewer trips to the store.** Rather than spending an hour per week shopping at the local supermarket, I only spend a few minutes, shopping there just for a few small, perishable items. Once every couple of months my husband accompanies me to a warehouse-type outlet where we make one large purchase of items such as laundry detergent, toilet paper, and meats (which we freeze). His help and a written shopping list makes the trip go faster. Because we now purchase less at the local supermarket, the trips there are relatively short and he is more inclined to help me out by picking up items on the way home from work. Between my husband's help and the warehouse outlet, I have cut down on the number of bladder-bouncing trips to the store in the car.

◆ **Don't be afraid to ask for help.** Needing help is nothing to be ashamed of. In the last century, barn-raising and home-building was a community effort and people often called on their neighbors to help them out. You'll find that many people are very helpful and compassionate if only you take the time to let them know you and know your situation. You may also make a new friend by confiding your illness. (After several years with both IC and fibromyalgia, I finally talked about it one day with my neighbor's grown son. Much to my surprise, I found that he too suffers from fibromyalgia). If you don't have room to store large-quantity food purchases for instance, but your neighbor has excess space, explain your situation and ask a neighbor if you can use some of the spare space at their house. If shopping is very difficult because of urinary frequency, a friend or relative may not mind picking up a few items now and then to save you a trip to the store.

◆ **Plan your trip at home and shop only with a list.** Janet, an IC sufferer of the past four years, says that frequency is her main problem. She needs to get in and out of the store quickly— not always an easy task. For her, a different strategy of many quick trips is most successful. She writes out her list in the order in which she goes through the aisles in the store. Her market is only a short distance from her house, and she finds that making several trips to the store per week means she purchases less per trip. She then always pays with cash so she can go through the express check-out line.

◆ **Use your computer to organize your shopping trip.** If you have a computer, some cooking and recipe software will print out a shopping list for you after you pick the recipes and meals for the week. (You can even set up one program, Mastercook, to print the list in the order in which you go down the aisles of your favorite store).

◆ **Shop during off-peak hours to get the task done quicker.** In general, supermarkets have the most business on Saturdays, around lunch time during the week, and in the late afternoon (as people stop by to pick up something on their way home from work). You can also ask the clerks at your favorite market, about the least crowded times. If you don't work outside the home, you can get through the lines faster by picking up groceries while most people are at their jobs. To avoid having to run to the market when it's crowded, keep supplies on hand for an "emergency dinner"— an easy to fix menu.

Meal preparation strategies

◆ **Cook once, eat twice.** Prepare twice as much food as you need for a dinner and freeze the rest. This is a strategy that works well for Barbra, who has had IC for over twenty years. She finds that soups, stews and casseroles usually freeze very well. So do muffins, breads and most cakes and some cookies. The frozen servings are helpful for those "flare" days when you don't feel like cooking. Barbra does most of her cooking this way and enjoys the time not spent in the kitchen, playing with her grandchildren.

◆ **Plan for leftovers.** For example, roast pork can be used later in the week to make a quick pork chop suey, so cook a larger roast than you need for one dinner.

◆ **Try one new recipe at a time.** New recipes often take a lot longer the first time you try them. You don't want to stand on your feet in the kitchen so long that you are in too much pain to enjoy the wonderful meal you've cooked.

◆ **Invest in yourself.** An investment in time-saving kitchen equipment is an investment in yourself. Food processors, slow cooking crock-pots, blenders, choppers, and microwave ovens can save a lot of time, and make clean-ups easier. A refrigerator with a larger freezer, or a stand-alone freezer may be a good investment for storing extra portions of IC-safe foods for the days when your symptoms at at their worst and you for those "flare days" when you absolutely can't cook. Purchase whatever you need to cut down on "on-your-feet" time in the kitchen.

◆ **Make your own convenience spice blends.** Store-bought blends of spices such as poultry seasoning, curry powder, or Chinese five-spice powder are easy to use, but expensive. They also may contain one spice that bothers a sensitive IC bladder. You may want to invest in a kitchen mortar and pestle (or one of those little coffee bean grinders), then grind and mix your own blends, storing them in airtight jars. If you do small tasks like this when you are feeling relatively good, you will reap enormous rewards on other days when you are hurting and can appreciate time-saving conveniences like IC-safe, pre-blended spice mixtures.

◆ **Enlist the aid of other people on a regular basis.** If you are the person in the family who has always done the cooking, think about switching chores with another family member. (My husband has become a wonderful chef of gourmet Chinese food. Although cooking felt strange at first, he found he liked the creativity involved, and welcomed the change from the numbers-oriented kind of work he did all day at the office.) Even an older child at home can start dinner by putting a casserole, potatoes, or roast in the oven. Don't be a martyr and refuse your family's help. Kids often enjoy being "grown-up" and helping out. Spouses can feel helpless in the face of your sudden illness. Helping in the kitchen gives your family an opportunity to do something constructive to ease the situation, as well as to show their love and appreciation of you. Think of preparing the meal as a family-together project, and these times may be the basis for many fond memories later.

◆ **Gradually introduce new foods to children.** If you are cooking IC-safe meals for the whole family, and will be changing the fare from what you've served in the past, don't serve too many new foods at once. Children like familiarity and won't appreciate a sudden and dramatic change. Try new IC-safe dishes on hassle-free nights when they are more likely to be in a good mood to try something new. Kids' favorites like spaghetti sauce and pepperoni pizza may be out for you. but not for them. They can still have their favorites if you freeze extra portions of IC-safe dishes that can be quickly reheated for you. Then go ahead and let the rest of the family enjoy their favorites.

Holidays and Entertaining

Stress, an inevitable part of the year-end holiday season, can make bladder symptoms worse. And when you feel bad, how can you enjoy celebrating? Here are three strategies that others with IC have tried:

◆ **Do the work once, enjoy the benefits year after year.** Plan menus ahead for holiday meals and "company dinners," complete with shopping lists. (Every year I save my menu, recipes, and shopping list for Christmas dinner in a notebook. After a few years I can recycle the same menu again and it will seem new). Practice any new recipes ahead of time so you won't be worn out, stressed out, and in pain instead of enjoying the occasion.

◆ **Give yourself a gift.** If you have traditionally cooked big meals and invited the family over for the holidays, consider giving yourself a gift of relaxation time. Start a new tradition of having everyone bring a dish, so there's less for you to cook. Or have a restaurant deliver some dishes (such as fancy desserts) that are time-consuming to make. You might also set aside one day during the absolute height of the hectic shopping season for "pampering"— taking a long hot bath, relaxing in front of the fireplace, watching TV— a day full of whatever relaxes and refreshes you. Mark it on your calendar and consider it an "appointment" with yourself that you must keep.

◆ **Make a plan to reduce holiday stress.** Take a few minutes, early in the season, to make a list of what tasks, events, and relationships are *really* important and emotionally satisfying to you. Then make a "guilt" list— those tasks you'd rather not do because they invariably make your bladder worse, yet you feel you just *have* to do them. See if you can reduce your participation in the tasks on the "guilt list" by asking other people to take a turn at doing soem of them, by paying someone else to do them, by putting some off until after the holiday season (when you are less stressed), or by just plain eliminating any unnecessary tasks. After all, will anyone really remember, five years from now, that you didn't dust under the bed this particular day?

◆ **Bake desserts you can't eat as individual portions.** When your guests leave after a holiday meal, do you find you have leftover portions of a luscious chocolate dessert you can't eat, lurking in your fridge and tempting you to "cheat"? One solution is to bake or cook those "forbidden" dishes in individual portions, making just enough for all the guests, with no leftovers. Bake several five-inch fruit tarts or turnovers rather than a pie. Even cakes can be baked as cupcakes, turned upside down, then frosted and decorated as individual little cakes. (Check party supply stores for very small novelty-shaped baking pans, too). The fewer of these delicious "no-no's" you have hanging around, the less you'll be tempted to eat them up... and pay later with a bladder flare. Just remember that smaller portions bake faster, so watch them closely.

A CLOSER LOOK AT SOME PROBLEM FOODS

Interstitial cystitis has no known cause, and has neither a cure nor a treatment that works for everyone. Yet it is human nature for us to be curious about things that affect us deeply. While the medical community continues to investigate possible causes, patients have little in the way of solid explanations for why they suffer from IC. People with IC yearn for answers and many of them spend considerable time educating themselves about their illness. One urologist remarked to his IC patient, Karen, that he was constantly amazed by the level of knowledge and motivation exhibited by his IC patients. Some people with IC search medical libraries and electronic databases for information on interstitial cystitis. Many look to support groups and telephone networks of other IC patients for hints and tips to help them gain control over their affliction.

The Interstitial Cystitis Association has found that on average, it takes five years for a patient to obtain a correct diagnosis of IC. By the time a diagnosis is finally obtained, he or she may have passed through many doctors' offices without obtaining a diagnosis or a treatment that helps. Sadly, this lengthy process can lead patients to become cynical and suspicious of doctors. IC support groups regularly see frustrated patients desperately seeking more information about their affliction— information they haven't received from their doctors. And one of the most common questions IC patients raise at support group meetings concerns diet.

At some time we've all asked, "Why do these particular foods cause me so much pain and frequency?" We harbor the hope that if we can just figure out what it is in the food that's causing a problem, then we can be more effective at avoiding it. Although medical knowledge of IC is expanding every year and new avenues of research are being opened, dietary factors have not been given much attention. It's too early for doctors to say for certain whether a few substances, out of the thousands in each food, are truly to blame. The medical community has, however, taken note of some of the chemical characteristics certain foods have in common— characteristics they suspect may contribute to our bladder symptoms.

Looking over the list of foods that trigger pain in IC bladders, doctors have pointed out that many of them are high in amine-type compounds such as tyramine, tyrosine, tryptophan, and phenylalanine. Many of these "trigger" foods are also quite acidic. Without going into great detail about complex chemical interactions, it's worthwhile to understand a few things about what these chemicals do in the body and why some people believe these substances may be responsible for the increases in symptom intensity that IC sufferers call "flares."

Some Substances in Foods

The nervous system is involved in many bodily functions, including the action of smooth muscles in the intestines, the circulatory system, and the bladder. The function of the nerves in the bladder, and the role of neurotransmitters which may affect them, have been the focus of much recent research on IC.

Neurotransmitters are substances which act in the body to facilitate communication between parts of the nervous system. They allow chemical messages to be transferred from one nerve cell to another. There are many neurotransmitters, and without them, pain signals would not get from the bladder to the brain, for instance.

Serotonin is one such neurotransmitter, and it figures prominently in sleep regulation, immune system function, emotional balance, blood flow, and pain control. The body makes serotonin from an amino acid, tryptophan. Tryptophan must be obtained from food, because the body cannot make it. Although no one is sure of the significance, it is curious that quite a few foods that IC patients find problematic, also have high levels of tryptophan. Cheddar cheese, bacon, and anchovies for instance, are all very high in this amino acid.

Histamine is familiar to most of us as the irritating substance that our sinuses produce when we have a cold or allergy attack, but it is also a neurotransmitter. A wide variety of foods that provoke IC bladders are high in histamine. (Many IC "trigger" foods contain high levels of histidine, an amino acid which can become histamine in the body). Red wine is particularly high in histamine. Anchovies, bacon and cheddar cheese are in fact "double whammy" foods— high in histamine as well as the serotonin precursor, tryptophan.

While there have been no scientific studies proving that the tryptophan or histamine in these foods cause bladder pain, there is evidence that histamine and sertoninin do play a role in IC. Two of the medications commonly used to treat IC, both affect histamine in the body. The prescription antihistamine hydroxyzine (sold under the trade names Atarax or Vistaril) and the histamine-blocker cimetidine (sold over-the-counter as Tagamet), are both used by many IC patients to combat their bladder pain. Some of the helpful IC medications affect the action of serotonin. The tricyclic antidepressant, amitriptyline, is a good example.

According to physician, professor of Pharmacology, and IC researcher Dr. T.C. Theoharides, hydroxyzine may also be effective for IC patients' migraines, irritable bowel syndrome, and allergies. Dr. Theoharides and others have done considerable research in the last fifteen years on the subject of mast cells and their involvement in interstitial cystitis, migraines, and irritable bowel syndrome (IBS). In one article published in 1997 in the medical journal *Urology*, it was noted that mast cells, which are often found in close proximity to nerve fibers in IC bladders, are also found close to nerve fibers in the colons of people with IBS. It is suspected that these mast cells are involved in producing the symptoms of both IC and IBS. Mast cells both produce histamine, and are triggered by histamine. The urine of IC patients has been found not only to be quite high in irritating histamine, but its break-down product, methylhistamine as well.

It is interesting to note that many people with IC find that their reactions to certain foods are much worse when they are under stress, and women with interstitial cystitis often note an increased sensitivity during certain times of the month. In a recently published study, Drs. Spanos, Pang, and colleagues found that in animals at least, psychological stress led to the activation of bladder mast cells. (I know that stress sure makes my bladder worse— but not at the time of the stress. There seems to be a delay of hours or even a day). Research with humans has found that female hormones, too, can activate bladder mast cells.

Three other chemicals, commonly found in foods that IC patients avoid, are tyramine, tyrosine, and phenylalanine. Tyramine is a monoamine and large amounts of it are found in red wine, aged cheeses, sour cream, soy sauce, anchovies, chocolate, avocadoes, and a few other food items that cause us bladder pain. According to Dr. Devin Starlanyl, a banana that is overripe can have quite a fair dose of tyramine too. In humans, tyramine causes effects similar to those caused by adrenaline, including the speeding up of the heart and the redirecting of blood flow.

Tyramine can also be produced by bacteria from an amino acid, tyrosine. Amino acids, such as tyrosine, are the building blocks of proteins. You may be sensitive to the tyramine formed in protein-rich foods that have been improperly stored, are slightly spoiled, or appear moldy. To avoid bacteria-formed tyramine as much as possible, dieticians recommend eating freshly prepared foods, and avoiding leftovers that have been stored quite awhile. Tyrosine is found in many of the foods that trouble IC sufferers, and it is a building block of several hormones produced by the thyroid and the adrenal glands.

Phenylalanine may be another amino acid important to consider, because it too, is high in some foods we avoid. Aspartame, for instance, is an artificial sweetener used in many dietetic and other food products and is notorious for causing bladder pain. Aspartame is metabolized in the body, and in the process, forms phenylalanine. Phenylalanine in turn can be converted to tyrosine in the body.

The list of foods high in tyramine and tyrosine is very similar to the list of foods that IC patients find are symptom-provoking. Because tyramine and tyrosine also affect certain aspects of the body's functioning, doctors suspect that these two substances may be involved in causing the bladder symptom flares which follow consumption of those foods.

But perhaps tryptophan, histamine, tyramine, and tyrosine still aren't the whole story. Mozzarella cheese (considered "safe" by many), is higher in all these substances than the notorious pain-provoker, cheddar cheese. Another interesting point is that pears and apples are about equal in the amounts of tyrosine, tryptophan, histamine and phenylalanine they contain. Yet pears seem to be "safe" while apples can be a problem for many people with IC. So why is it that apples and cheddar can cause a big flare while mozzarella and pears don't? Acidity seems to be another factor that correlates with whether or not a food causes a flare in bladder symptoms. (Apples are more acidic than pears, and cheddar is more acidic than mozzarella.)

When you are concerned with acidity, it is important be familiar with the "pH" scale. The term pH means "potential of hydrogen" and it is a measure of the acidity or alkalinity of anything. The numbers on the pH scale range from 1 to 14. The smaller numbers are acid and the larger ones are basic (or alkaline). A pH of 7 is neutral. As a non-scientist, I find it's easier to remember that the bigger the number the more alkaline it is, by thinking of the saying "bigger is better."

People with IC sometimes think that their urine must be "acid," because it often feels "hot" when they urinate and when they aren't urinating, their urethra has a burning sensation that can feel as if acid is being poured through it. Many years ago Larrian Gillespie, in her book *You Don't Have to Live with Cystitis!* (Rawson Associates, 1986) reported that the urine of IC sufferers was typically alkaline. But more recently urologist and IC researcher Dr. Kristene Whitmore, in a book she wrote with Rebecca Chalker titled *Overcoming Bladder Disorders* (Harper and Row, 1990) noted that other urologists have found that IC patients' urine is actually quite variable, and like that of most healthy people, it can be either slightly acidic or slightly alkaline.

Without guidance from knowledgeable doctors, and in the absence of much research on foods and interstitial cystitis, some ingenious IC sufferers have attempted to sort out what foods to avoid by measuring the acidity of their urine with litmus or nitrazine paper after they eat. Another strategy some people have tried is following a diet based on whether the food produces "acid ash" or "alkaline ash" in the urine. To date, there has been no scientific study indicating these procedures are really useful to patients.

When you eat food, the digestive tract breaks the food down into smaller chemical units, extracts what it needs, and lets the remainder pass through as waste. The substances it retains fuel the body's many chemical reactions. Those reactions use up fuel from food much like a fire in your fireplace "uses up" the logs. And much like the logs, there is an "ash" leftover— the stuff that doesn't "burn" (in the body's case, a chemical "burn"). What's left of the nutrients in foods after the body uses them, is referred to as "ash" too. Whether the ash is alkaline or acid depends on the types of chemicals left over. Some foods leave an acid waste product ("acid ash"), and some leave an alkaline waste product ("alkaline ash"). This ash waste product needs to be removed from the body to prevent a buildup, which is called acidosis or alkalosis. One way to get rid of the ash is in urine.

When an ash contains predominantly sulfur, phosphorus or chlorine, it is acidic. Foods with a lot of protein, such as meat, fish, and eggs are generally acid-ash forming. Cereals can also be acid-ash. Cranberries form an acid ash in the body, and they will turn the urine acid. (People with kidney or bladder stones are told by doctors to eat foods that form an acid ash. The stones are alkaline, so they will dissolve in the acidic urine caused by eating foods like meat and fish).

Other foods form an alkaline ash, and can turn the urine alkaline. Milk, for instance, leaves an alkaline ash. Citrus fruit also forms an alkaline ash. Citric acid is metabolized by the body, and since it is used up, it does not turn the urine acid. Thus, even though citrus fruit goes into the body as a very acidic substance, it makes the urine more alkaline. It is interesting that though cranberries produce an acid ash, and citrus produces an alkaline ash, both cause bladder pain in people with IC. I've found that trying to follow a diet based on whether the "ash" is acid, won't be of much help. But when a food we eat is acid to the taste buds, and acid as it hits the stomach, watch out—it could cause a symptom flare.

Some IC sufferers also try to maintain their bodily fluids as slightly acidic or slightly alkaline in the belief that it will affect the growth of various organisms, and therefore their IC pain. There is no conclusive evidence yet that IC is caused by a particular organism, although many investigators have tried unsuccessfully to find one that may be responsible. Some studies have noted that IC patients have more organisms in their bladders than healthy controls, but one predominant organism was not found, and the significance of the bacterial population in IC bladders is uncertain. Investigation into the possible role of bacteria in IC is ongoing. (Quite a few IC sufferers I have talked to, though, do say that their bladders seem overly sensitive to even low levels of bacteria, becoming more painful long before there are enough organisms in the urine to test positive for an oncoming bladder infection).

Another tactic that some IC patients have tried, is a low-sodium diet. They believe that if salt, which is sodium chloride, irritates a fresh wound on the skin, then sodium in various foods must do the same to their irritated bladder. There is no scientific evidence that a low-sodium diet is helpful for controlling bladder pain in IC patients, or that products with sodium in them should not be consumed because they irritate the lining of an IC bladder. (One treatment that doctors often use for IC, involves putting heparin sodium in direct contact with the bladder, and many people with IC find that taking a bit of baking soda (sodium bicarbonate) in water, helps with bladder pain triggered by eating something acid). Until doctors have conclusive evidence of a role for sodium in exacerbating IC symptoms, I don't bother with restricting my sodium intake.

If you have severe frequency however, you may want to avoid eating large quantities of salty foods because you will then be quite thirsty and consume more water. The increased water intake may in turn result in more trips to the bathroom. On the other side of the coin, those who have a lot of pain sometimes find that drinking ample water during the day, helps. They feel that "flushing" the bladder or "diluting the urine" is an advantage for them. Sound arguments can be made for both drinking lots of water, and avoiding too much water. With regard to salty foods and water intake, each person has to experiment and find what works best for him or her.

One other phenomenon that some IC patients have noticed, is that sugary foods, when eaten immediately before bedtime, cause them more pain and frequency the next morning. They find that eating a protein-rich food (such as roast beef, tuna, or cottage cheese) before bed is much better than, say, ice cream. If this situation describes you, then you may also benefit from eating several small meals throughout the day, rather than a couple large ones, and making sure that each meal has some protein-rich food. Several IC patients I know find they are helped by limiting their intake of sugary foods, especially avoiding sweets alone, when consumed without any protein-rich food. Some people have benefitted by following the low-carbohydrate diet suggested by Dr. Barry Sears in his book, *The Zone* (Harper Collins, 1995). Again, this phenomenon is a very individual thing, so experimentation is crucial.

Now that we have taken a general look at some of the suspect substances that naturally occur in food, there is one more category of dietary items worth mentioning: food additives. There are more than 2,000 food additives in use today and they include flavor enhancers, preservatives, colorants, sweeteners and many other chemicals put in our food. Some of these are put in the food solely for the convenience or profit of the manufacturer, distributor, or retailer. From a consumer's point of view they may seem totally unnecessary. Other additives though, are there to protect consumers from contamination and food poisoning. Regardless of their purpose for being there, some additives, according to the American Academy of Allergy, Asthma, and Immunology (AAAAI), cause adverse reactions in susceptible people.

You may find that certain food additives will cause a flare in your bladder pain, urgency, or frequency. Because so many people with IC have allergies, it is unclear so far whether our reactions to these additives represent an expression of an allergy, or are a part of the process of IC. Either way, since allergies/intolerances are very individual and so are the food reactions of people with IC, you will have to experiment with various products and keep good records to figure out which, if any, cause trouble for you. Here are some additives that the AAAAI list as problematic for susceptible people: benzoates (including sodium and potassium benzoate), BHA, BHT, FD&C dyes (particularly yellow #5), MSG (monosodium glutamate), nitrates and nitrites, parabens, and sulfites.

Artificial additives in canned and bottled foods are easy to spot because they are listed on the label, but other foods where you may not suspect additives are: fresh shrimp, mushrooms, shredded dried coconut, and dried fruit. These may be treated with sulfites, the most common of which is sodium metabisulfite. (Wash the shrimp and mushrooms well, and carefully scrutinize labels on the other items. Untreated dried coconut and fruit is available. See Appendix B). Wines often have low levels of natural sulfites which occur as part of the winemaking process, but some wineries add more. If you boil off the alcohol, the sulfites may not be a problem for you because heat degrades them. If you're still concerned, you can buy wine for cooking that doesn't have added sulfites. (See Appendix B for places that carry such products).

Simple Tricks to Head Off A Flare

We all tend to "cheat" now and then, eating foods that we know will cause problems later. But don't we deserve a little enjoyment? Sure! Sometimes, mercifully, our bladder lets us get away with it. Other times we aren't so lucky.

If the food we've eaten is acid, sometimes the horrible symptom flare that follows can be averted by taking a buffering product. In my experience, this works well to counteract the acidity of foods such as salad dressing or fruit, but won't work as well on non-acid foods whose main drawback is tyramine or histamine. (Buffers are chemicals that protect the acid-base balance of something else because they can combine with an acid or a base).

A teaspoon of baking soda in a glass of water is one popular tactic that uses a bicarbonate buffer. If you have high blood pressure or a heart condition, check with your doctor before using baking soda. Tums (a calcium carbonate buffer) is also very popular, though the calcium can cause constipation in some people, particularly if taken in large amounts.

A new non-prescription product on the market, called Prelief, is being marketed as a dietary supplement useful for combatting the effects of eating acid foods. Barbra, a long-time IC sufferer, was very enthusiastic about her experience with Prelief. "This works so much better for me than the Tums. One little pill and I can eat things like salad dressing again!" The manufacturer claims it "works on the food, not on you," but doctors at the University of California at Berkeley, School of Public Health, put the product to the test and found otherwise. They tested Prelief's acid-reducing power on lemon, orange, tomato and apple juices, as well as on coffee and water. When used as the manufacturer recommends, it had virtually no effect on the acidity of any of the water or fruit juices, but did have a minor effect on the acidity of the coffee. (Prelief is calcium glycerophosphate. Its lack of effect is not surprising, since phosphates usually acidify substances). So, does it help IC patients? Well, some are people are helped and others aren't. No one knows why this happens, but the phenomenon is being investigated.

Some IC sufferers find they can't take vitamin C (ascorbic acid) supplements in any form, but others find that a buffered version doesn't bother their bladder. Buffered vitamin C products usually contain calcium carbonate, the same thing that is in Tums. Lisa, a young mother of an active one-year-old, finds that antacids like Tums only seem to help her IC symptoms if taken while eating acid foods, or very soon after. "If I get busy and have to wait an hour or so before taking the antacid, then I'm in trouble... once the pain gets going and I'm running to the bathroom every five minutes, it's too late. But if I take it right after eating something, then I'm usually okay, " she says.

For me, anything that reduces stomach acidity also helps my bladder, and anything that increases it makes my bladder worse. Tagamet (which reduces stomach acid by blocking the action of histamine) sometimes helps me, and I have heard from others who have tried similar products with successful results. Like Lisa's experience with the antacids, though, I found timing is important. These products are most helpful for *my* IC pain if taken before dinner or at bedtime. Your experience may be different. Be sure to consider the timing of the dose when you evaluate whether or not an acid-buffer or histamine-blocker helps you eat certain foods. Also check with your doctor and/or pharmacist before using buffers or histamine blockers, because these can adversely affect certain prescription medications. Now let's look at a few problem foods in particular, and what we can do to avoid or overcome their effects.

Cheese

When milk or cream is made into cheese, it undergoes chemical changes that alter the amounts of some substances, and convert others into new compounds. When the cheese ages or "ripens," it goes through even more chemical changes that alter its taste and character. The longer a cheese ages, the sharper it tastes. While this may be good news for the taste buds, it's definitely bad news for IC bladders.

The ripening process does several things to cheese, all of which may play a role in causing bladder pain. First, ripened cheeses are higher in histamine, a substance that affects mast cells and can cause allergic or gastrointestinal symptoms in some people. Doctors believe that bladder mast cells may play a role in IC symptoms.

Not only are ripened cheeses high in histamine, they are quite acidic as well. Cheese-makers need to control the acidity and prevent unwanted bacterial contamination of the ripened cheese, so they will often add acids such as citric acid or fumaric acid to the cheese. While these strong acids may control bacteria in the cheese, they can cause symptom flares for people with IC. To make matters worse, ripened cheeses such as cheddar, parmesan or brie are also high in tyramine, another substance that may aggravate sensitive IC bladders.

Some cheeses do not go through the ripening process, so are considered "safer" for people with IC. The following cheeses are considered "unripened:"

Cottage cheese
Cream cheese
Farmer cheese
Feta
Gjetost
Gournay (often sold in the U.S. under the name "Boursin")
Marscapone
Mozzarella
Muenster
Neufchatel
Pot cheese
Ricotta
Scamorze

Not everyone with IC may be able to eat all of these "safer" cheeses, though. Those with IBS, a sensitivity to lactic acid (acidophilus) bacteria, an allergy to cow's milk, or a lactose intolerance may have problems with some or all of them. Be sure to check the labels carefully for any preservatives, too. Some otherwise "safe" cheese products have added benzoates, a substance which causes problems for many allergic individuals, as well as those with interstitial cystitis.

Some people with IC may be able to eat Monterey jack cheese. It is ripened, but just barely. Whereas many cheeses are ripened for months, jack is only allowed to ripen about two weeks. (Don't confuse this cheese with something called "hard jack." Hard jack is Monterey jack cheese that has fully ripened and become a hard, aged cheese that will likely cause a symptom flare).

Another cheese product that some people with IC say they can tolerate is Velveeta or American cheese. Typically, these type of products have at least some aged cheddar-type cheese in them. It is a small amount and unless you are very sensitive to cheddar it may be worth trying. Lori, an IC sufferer of about three years, uses Velveeta in many of the foods that she used to make with cheddar. She says that most of her recipes are easy to adapt, her husband and kids don't mind the change, and her bladder is a lot happier now.

Coffee

My daughter is in college now, and drives a time-weathered little car that she has plastered with bumper stickers. The most prominent one declares her attitude toward coffee— that favorite beverage of college students doing late-night cram sessions. It proclaims, "death before decaf."

I too, used to think that way about coffee— the stronger the better. Nothing like a good jolt of caffeine to get the blood flowing and the heart pumping in the morning! Now that I have IC and rarely drink coffee, I find I miss more than just the taste of it. I miss that wake-up effect when I need to be alert for night driving. I miss sharing a post-meeting cup of coffee with co-workers. I miss the romantic interludes my husband and I used to share over capuccinos and chocolate cheesecake.

I've come to understand a big part of why those of us with IC are so reluctant to forego coffee— coffee drinking is a part of the American social fabric. We all want to fit in, be accepted, and participate in the things everyone else does. So sometimes when I'm with other people, I just order decaf and hope for the best.

In talking to other people with IC, it seems we all agree that caffeine content is not the only problem with coffee. Very acid coffee can also trigger symptom flares. Curiously, it seems that some of us are more sensitive to the caffeine, while others are most sensitive to the acidity. And because we are all different, some of us can drink any kind of coffee and others have to stay away from even the tiniest amounts in any form. Experimentation is the best way to find your pattern of sensitivity and level of tolerance for coffee.

Caffeine

In terms of caffeine, brewed coffee packs a real punch— 80 to 120 mg of caffeine per cup, whereas tea when brewed averages only around 45 mg of caffeine per cup. (Most cola beverages only have about 30 mg of caffeine per 8-ounce cup). Two of the most important factors affecting the caffeine content of a cup of coffee are the type of beans used, and the brewing method.

There are three varieties of coffee beans that are commercially grown: C. arabica, C. liberica, and C. robusta. The arabica beans are thought of as the highest quality and are the most widely used beans in the United States. Liberica beans are considered inferior and are rarely sold in North America. Robusta beans, though very popular in Italy, are considered to be of inferior quality here and are mostly used in cheaper blends. Robusta beans are used in the pre-ground canned coffee you find at the supermarket.

The caffeine content of the beans can vary depending on where they are grown. On the whole however, the robusta beans have from 2 to 2½ times the amount of caffeine as the arabicas. (Remember this when comparing canned coffee to "gourmet" coffee beans, even if both are labeled "98 percent caffeine-free"). Most coffee beans imported from Africa are robustas. Also be aware that the Extra-Medellin variety, cultivated in Columbia, is among the most highly caffeinated in the world. (There is one curious species of coffee plant that grows caffeine-free beans. It is found on Grand Comoro, an island near Madagascar, off the eastern coast of Africa. Unfortunately, those rare beans aren't commercially available).

Caffeine is readily absorbed by the body and reaches peak levels in about an hour, though this rate can vary from one individual to another. Women generally metabolize caffeine faster than men. Though you can't change nature, you may be able to slow down the speed with which the caffeine is absorbed by eating some food with your coffee.

Decaf coffees are very popular among those with IC who drink coffee. Coffee can be decaffeinated in several ways. The two most often-used methods involve either treating the coffee with chemicals that bind to the caffeine and remove it, or simply washing the coffee with water, a process that dissolves the water-soluble caffeine.

A number of years ago the FDA prohibited the use of a certain decaffeinating chemical due to its cancer-causing potential. Other less dangerous chemicals are now used and limits are set on any possible residue left in the coffee. Some U.S. companies find it cheaper to export their beans for chemical decaffeination. The FDA checks the beans for traces of chemicals when they come back into the country. Residues of only a few parts per million can cause the agency to refuse the re-entry of an entire lot of beans.

Because of health and safety concerns about chemical extraction, water process decaffeination has become popular. The water process, however, also washes away some of the sugars and delicate substances that give the coffee flavor.

A third, though rarely used, process for caffeine removal is by carbon dioxide. This is a very expensive method. It is regarded as the best method of removing caffeine though, because it removes it without chemicals and leaves other flavor-imparting substances intact.

Another factor affecting the amount of caffeine in a cup of coffee is the brewing method. Some people with IC say they can tolerate espresso better than drip-brewed coffee, and this may be because espresso has considerably less caffeine. In making espresso, a smaller amount of water is in contact with the ground coffee beans for a shorter length of time. As a result, less of the beans' water-soluble caffeine is dissolved. For much the same reason, you may also find that drip-brewed coffee is more bladder-friendly than percolated coffee.

Decaf coffees have around 1 to 6 mg of caffeine per cup— around 95 to 98 percent less than regular coffee. And, if you prefer your coffee with chicory, don't worry about added caffeine from the chicory. The chicory adds color and body but no caffeine.

Coffee acidity

I've found that the acidity of coffee is another factor that influences whether or not it will cause bladder symptoms. Two kinds of acids in particular make coffee more bitter tasting: trigonelline and chlorogenic acids. If you have gastrointestinal problems, be aware that these two also make coffee less digestible and may cause "sour stomach." Tannic acid, also called tannin, is a known bladder irritant and is responsible for staining teeth. Coffee has a high level of tannin, as does tea. (Try drinking your coffee through a straw, if you want to minimize tooth-staining).

There are three main factors that control the amount of acids in the coffee you drink. The first factor is the type of bean. Some beans are just naturally more acidic than others. Yemen Mocha beans for instance, are naturally very acidic. On the other hand, coffee beans from the Indonesian islands, such as Java and Sumatra, are very mild and much less acidic. Jamaican Blue Mountain is another coffee I've found that is very mild and low-acid. (It is very expensive when you can find it, and not available year-round. Most of the crop is exported to Japan each year).

Another factor affecting the acidity of coffee is the roasting process. Green coffee beans have no flavor. It is the roasting process that brings out the aromatic oil, called caffeol, which gives coffee its flavor. Roasting is a complex process. While it imparts a characteristic flavor to the beans, numerous chemical reactions inside the bean are involved. The time and temperature of roasting is critical. Roasting is considered an art as well as a science, and each company has a preferred roasting technique.

In general though, roasting will lessen the chemical acidity of the coffee beans. The more lightly roasted the coffee, the lighter in color and more acid they are. Beans which are very dark brown and shiny have been roasted longer and are the best bet for a low-acid cup of coffee. (When people talk about coffee bitterness and acidity, they may not be referring to the chemical nature of the brew. "Acidity" and "bitterness" are terms used by coffee connoisseurs in describing the taste of the coffee. It is the chemical acidity, the "pH", that IC patients need to be concerned with. When talking to a coffee vendor, be sure they know you mean chemical acidity when you ask about low-acid coffees).

Brewing method can affect the acidity of coffee, too. Hot water tends to bring out the acids in coffee. Eliot Jordan, of Peet's Coffee and Tea, suggests this method to make a low-acid cup of coffee: since it is heat in brewing that extracts the acids, simply steep a half pound of ground coffee in a quart of cold water overnight. Then strain the liquid out to make a thick concentrate (straining may take an hour or more). Measure two ounces into a mug, then add six ounces boiling water to make hot coffee. According to Eliot Jordan, "It might not be the best tasting cup, but it is low acid."

One person with IC posted a message on an internet newsgroup saying she can drink coffee again on a regular basis, but only if she uses that "cold concentrate" brewing method. Containers specially designed for making coffee from concentrate are marketed by Toddy and a couple of other manufacturers, but you don't need to buy such special equipment. There are a few difficulties to watch out for in making coffee this way, though. (See my recipe and notes on storage in Part Two, Miscellaneous, page 186).

The effect of storage

After roasting, the delicate oils in the coffee beans are sensitive to oxygen and storage temperature. If stored too long or in a warm place, they will oxidize and turn rancid. Cool temperature keeps them fresher, longer. For the freshest, best-tasting cup of coffee, keep your beans (whole or already ground) in the refrigerator but don't freeze them. Freezing coffee beans will destroy the delicate natural oils and flavor.

Another tip: you've no doubt noticed that coffee tends to get stronger tasting after it's left standing awhile, or is reheated over and over. Be sure to remove the filter and grounds the minute your pot of drip-brewed coffee or percolated coffee is done. The last bit of coffee dripping from the grounds is the strongest in terms of caffeine. You may find that your bladder is happier when you drink only fresh-brewed coffee.

Coffee suppliers

If you are fortunate enough to be able to tolerate a little coffee, experiment with different types of coffee and brewing methods to find out what works for you. You may find that say, Java beans from one company, irritate your bladder more than Java beans from another company. This could be due to any number of factors, so be sure to try different brands, too.

One way to insure that you get the least-caffeinated and least-acidic cup of coffee possible, is to buy roasted beans and grind them yourself. Small electric coffee grinders can be bought for $25 or less. Some supermarkets now carry unground beans, or you can shop at local specialty stores and national coffee-shop chains like Starbucks or Gloria Jean's. Another option is to mail-order your beans, but they may be a bit more expensive that way. There are many mail-order coffee suppliers but here are two of my favorites:

◆ *Diedrich Coffee*

This company uses the carbon dioxide method of decaffeination (regarded as the best method in the industry) and also has low-acid beans available year-round in a decaf version. They have been in the custom roasting and importing business since 1912. You can get information or order by phone at (800) 354-5282. They also have recently set up a site on the internet (http://www.diedrich.com). My personal favorites for low-acid, low-caffeine coffee are their Decaf Java and Decaf Sumatra.

◆ *Peet's Coffee and Tea*

Peet's is popular on the West Coast and has been around a long time, but is a bit smaller operation than Diedrich. Call for information or to order ground or whole beans at: (800)-999-2132. Of their coffees, I prefer Decaf Sumatra.

Sue, who has had both IC and vulvodynia for several years, has found another source of coffee that she finds to be "safe" for her bladder. She's also enthused about other products the company offers. "I am delighted to be able to drink coffee again as I miss so many beverages I can no longer tolerate. I can drink a cup of their decaf coffee on an empty bladder without pain. They also have a tasty decaf coffee extract you can mix with vanilla powder for a yummy drink." Here's more information on Sue's favorite coffee supplier:

◆ *The Coffee Bean & Tea Leaf*

This company imports and grinds their own coffee for a chain of stores. If you live near one of their stores, you can drop in and try a cup of decaf coffee before you purchase beans or ground coffee. Their home office is in Camarillo, California and from there they will send beans by mail to any part of the country. (Call 1-800-832-5323 to order, or for more information). The staff is very helpful and they will even send samples with your order. At the moment a pound of coffee runs about $9.75, but Sue says, "It's well worth it for the quality and flavor."

Coffee Substitutes

If all else fails, or you have a more severe case of IC, you may want to try one of the grain-based beverages such as Pero, Cafix, or Postum. They are dark like coffee, and taste somewhat like coffee, but have no caffeine. Many are made from barley. These products get mixed reviews from IC patients. Most people find they cause no bladder problems, but a few say they will definitely cause a flare.

Of the coffee substitutes I tried, I thought Natural Touch's "Roma" tasted the closest to coffee. Thankfully, it didn't cause me any bladder pain or frequency either. I also tried mixing the Roma with a little low-acid decaf coffee to improve the taste. Supermarkets occasionally carry coffee substitutes, but you're more likely to find them at a specialty market. (See Appendix B for some markets that carry several brands of grain-based coffee substitutes).

Wine & Beer

In a mast cell disease, the mast cells become sensitized and small amounts of histamine can then provoke the sensitized cells to cause symptoms. Although the role of mast cells in IC hasn't been completely explored, recent research shows that at least some IC patients may have bladder mast cell abnormalities. For this reason, people with IC may want to avoid consuming things that have a lot of histamine.

There are a number of common foods from which you can get a large dose of histamine, and many of them are ones that people with IC say cause them increased pain and frequency. These include aged cheeses, hard-cured sausages, pickled cabbage, and anchovies, among others. But the most troubling histamine-containing items are likely to be wine and beer. These two deliver a double punch— first they unload a dose of irritating histamine, then the alcohol interferes with the action of a histamine-destroying enzyme. When the enzyme can't break down the obnoxious histamine, the body suffers a histamine build-up.

Wine

If you have IC and have tried drinking wine lately, chances are it was a white wine. Even a small amount of red wine provokes excruciating bladder symptoms in large numbers of IC patients, while some white wines are often tolerable. If you are sensitive to histamine, the reason is simple. Red wines have 20 to 200 times more histamine than white wines. In terms of histamine content, red wines head the list, with champagnes, sparkling wines, and beer coming in a close second. White wines have the lowest histamine content of the wines and beers.

Of course, histamine is not the only constituent of wine that may cause problems for people with IC. Besides histamine, other problematic substances in wine are: alcohol, various acids, tyramine and tyrosine, sulfites, and certain additives it may also contain.

The more alcohol in the wine, the longer it takes for the alcohol (and therefore the histamine) to be removed from the body. Some wines have more alcohol than others as a natural result of the fermentation process. Typically most wines will have around 9% to 14% alcohol. Certain dessert wines such as sherries are deliberately fortified with even more alcohol. Vermouth, muscatel, angelica, California tokay, white port and tawny port can have as much as 21% alcohol.

Wine is also very acidic by nature, and a certain amount of acidity is considered a desirable quality by vintners. If the grapes are not acidic enough, winemakers will add citric acid, malic acid and/or tartaric acid to supplement the grapes' natural amounts of these. Most white wines are around 0.5% to 0.7% acid, with champagnes often being a very high 0.75% acid. Dessert wines, though high in alcohol, are fairly low in acid compared to the white table wines. The following chart compares the alcohol and acidity some of the various kinds of white table wines and dessert wines.

WHITE TABLE & DESSERT WINES

Acidity	**Alcohol**	**Wine**
Very High	High	Champagne, sparkling wines
High	Low-Med	Riesling
High	Varies	Chenin Blanc
Med-High	High	Pinot Blanc
Med	Med	Muscat
Med	Low-Med	Muller-Thurgau
Med-Low	High	Chardonnay
Med-Low	High	Pinot Gris
Low	Very High	Gewurztraminer
Low	Med	Semillon
Low	Very High	Cream Sherry, Vermouth, Tokay, White Port, Tawny Port

For IC patients, unfortunately, this is a case where you can't have it all. Good luck finding a white wine that is both low-acid *and* low-alcohol. To make the picture grimmer, there is the matter of additives to consider. Sulfites are sometimes used in winemaking to control unwanted organisms that may contaminate the wine. (This is the same chemical that restaurants use to prevent the leafy greens at salad bars from turning brown). Most wine naturally contains a little of these compounds (dry, white wines have the least), but when large amounts are added to wine or to food it can cause allergic symptoms in some people, and may cause bladder pain for those of us with IC. Sulfites are rarely used any more by commercial winemakers, but very small wineries or cheap imported wines may contain a considerable amount of sulfites. Fortunately for us, Federal law requires all wines sold in the U.S., which have sulfites added, to be labelled as such.

One more item often used as a preservative in cheap wines, potassium sorbate, may adversely affect some people. It is also found in some soft drinks and other products. Usually potassium sorbate is not found in the better wines because when they are stored for any length of time, the potassium sorbate causes an off-flavor to develop.

So what are IC patients to do? First, most everyone with IC stays away from red wines, which in addition to having a huge amount of irritating histamine, have tyramine, a fair amount of acid, and plenty of alcohol. (I can get away with a little sherry now and then if my bladder is having a "good day," but even the tiniest amount of red wine sets my bladder on an awful rampage). Champagnes and sparkling wines, being quite acidic, are also problematic.

Whether or not you are able to drink any other white or dessert wine may be an individual matter. One IC patient I know can drink a low-acid white dessert wine, but not a higher acid (but lower alcohol) Chardonnay. Other IC patients I have talked to can't tolerate drinking any kind of wine. Cooking with sherry or low-acid white wines is often the only way some IC patients can consume alcoholic beverages.

In my experience it seems to be the acidity more than the alcohol in white wines that causes me bladder problems. Using a buffer, such as baking soda or Tums, helps if I have to drink a bit of white wine. Taking some food with it, especially an alkaline food like the soda crackers used for hors d'oeuvres, seems to slow down the impact for me. But by all means, experiment and see what works for you. Be careful too, if you take prescription medications, especially painkillers. They may interact dangerously with alcohol.

Sherry is low-acid and can often be used in baking or cooking. Alcohol boils at a lower temperature than water, so the heat evaporates it. Also, I try to buy a moderately priced sherry rather than a cheap one, in order to avoid added preservatives. (Check Appendix B for some places that sell wines that do not have added sulfites). Sulfites, which may be in cheap cooking sherry (check the label) are theoretically destroyed by the heat of cooking. However, I've found that baking with other products listing sodium metabisulfite (the form of sulfite put in the cheap wines) has resulted in severe bladder flares for me. I wonder if perhaps the heat of baking may not have been enough to destroy all the sulfites. At any rate, I now check labels very carefully and have never had a bladder symptom flare as a result of cooking with a moderately priced sherry that doesn't list any preservatives or added sulfites on the label.

Beer

Like wine, beer contains some histamine and also alcohol, which can impair the body's ability to get rid of the histamine. The alcohol content varies widely from around 2% by volume to around 12% by volume. Most beers however, are in the 4-6% range. In general, Belgian and French ales, Stout ales, Bock lagers, and flavored beers have a greater alcohol content than others.

"Lite" beers or "near beers" have less alcohol than regular beer. Alcohol content in beer can also vary depending on laws of the State in which you live. I will never forget the time I was about twenty-two and moved from California, a state with low-alcohol beer, to New Jersey, where the same brand of beer packed a substantially bigger alcoholic wallop. It didn't take me long to find out why my friends were twittering and chuckling to themselves as I naively drank my first glass of New Jersey beer. It hit me like a freight train and I was under the table in no time.

Besides avoiding wine and beer altogether, is there anything we can do to lessen the bladder symptoms brought on by an occasional alcoholic drink? Possibly. Evelyn Tribole, a registered dietician, suggests that a diet low in vitamin B-6 may aggravate a food histamine problem. Vitamin B-6, she says, is crucial for the enzyme activity that helps rid the body of histamine, and eating food high in vitamin B-6 immediately before ingesting alcohol may help. Good sources of vitamin B-6 are meat, fish, poultry, sunflower seeds, corn, and whole grains. (You may have an unexpectedly negative reaction though, to the vitamin B-6 supplements commonly sold in drugstores and health food stores. See Appendix A).

Tomatoes

Acidity is the main reason most people with IC give for not eating tomatoes, although they can contain a small amount of tyramine too. But if we avoid them altogether, we miss out on the fiber, the vitamins and minerals, and the natural antioxidants, not to mention the delicious taste. I know I sure miss a good, thick, tomatoey spaghetti sauce. Some fortunate people have found that they can eat small amounts of fresh tomatoes, as slices on a sandwich for instance, but not stewed tomatoes or canned tomato sauces. Some IC sufferers with a green thumb have also found that they can have a little of the less-acidic fruits (such as tomatoes), but only if they grow it themselves. Unfortunately, some of us with IC have bladders so sensitive we cannot eat any kind of tomatoes, in any amount or form.

No one knows for sure why tomatoes are such a problem and IC sufferers have such a variable response to them. But if we look at how tomatoes get from field to table, we find some reasons why we may need to approach tomatoes with caution, and some factors we may be able to control enough to be able to eat tomatoes.

First we need to realize that growers plant the tomato varieties that are most economically beneficial to them, and that is usually a tomato variety that sprouts quickly, is resistant to plant disease, and has fruit that won't fall apart during shipping. After harvest, if the tomatoes are not going to be canned, they are sold to various buyers and distributors of fresh produce. When supermarkets buy tomatoes, they look for ones with "eye appeal", tomatoes that are round and firm and unblemished. According to one supermarket produce manager, consumers in the U.S. are very picky about the appearance of their fruit and vegetables and will buy only what looks perfect on the outside. But the tomato variety that is a botanical bonanza for the grower, or a beauty queen in the produce section, may also be very acidic. Different varieties of the same fruit or vegetable can have quite different average levels of acidity, and the low-acid varieties may not show up in your supermarket. Some of the least acid tomato varieties have fruit that look "funny" because of their odd-ball skin coloration or tendency to have blemishes. Some don't ship well. But the lower-acid varieties are delicious, healthful, and a lot of IC sufferers can eat them with little or no problem. If acidity is the main reason tomatoes bother you, try lower acid varieties.

Those with IC have more problems with canned tomatoes than fresh, and it's no wonder. According to agricultural expert Dr. Timothy Hartz of the University of California, Davis, many growers who plant their tomato crops for commercial canning actually want an acid tomato. They want to grow an acid tomato because the canners they sell to find acidity in tomatoes desirable. Acid helps ensure that the tomato product won't spoil before the consumer can use it, so in order to be commercially canned, tomatoes have to have a certain level of acidity. If the tomatoes don't have it, the canners have to buy an acid, such as citric acid, and add it to the tomatoes during processing. Citric acid, because it is considered by the Federal government to be a "GRAS" (Generally Recognized As Safe) substance, may not show up on the can's label. Some brands of tomato paste, for instance, list "natural flavor" on the label. That vague term may represent something which contains monosodium glutamate, citric acid, or another bladder-provoking substance. "Natural flavor" is a catch-all term, so approach products listing it on the label, with caution.

The grow-your-own alternative

Some people with IC have found that they can have all the tomatoes they want, if the tomatoes are low-acid varieties they grow in their back yard. Luckily, there are still some of the older open-pollinated low-acid varieties of tomato around. There are also a few hybrid varieties which are lower in acid. But what is meant by "low-acid"? And how do the low-acid tomatoes rate in comparison to other foods?

The following chart shows the approximate relative acidity of some common foods. Remember that acidity or alkalinity is measured on a "pH" scale, where a pH of 1 is very acid, a pH of 7 is neutral, and a pH of 14 is very alkaline). The pH scale is logarithmic, which means that a pH of 2 is ten times more acid than a pH of 3. This means that a soft drink can have 100 times the acidity of a fairly acid tomato. (It's something to think about when taking an antacid). Looking closely at the range of values for tomatoes and doing a little calculation, we find that a tomato with a pH of 4.5, for instance, is only about half as acid as one with a pH of 4.1.

Food	Acidity (in pH)
Lime juice	1.8 to 2.0
Most soft drinks	2.0 to 4.0
Vinegars	2.4 to 3.4
Grapefruit	3.0 to 3.3
Peaches	3.4 to 3.6
Grapes	3.0 to 4.0
Tomatoes	4.0 to 4.5
Carrots	4.9 to 5.3
Peas	5.8 to 6.4
Milk	6.3 to 6.6
Eggs	7.6 to 8.0

While for some people, the lower acidity of one tomato over another may not make any difference, for others, it may mean the ability to eat at least some tomatoes. Looking again at the list, we can see that tomatoes are pretty much a "borderline" food as far bladder symptoms go. Foods above tend to be problematic, and foods below are generally regarded as safe.

If you grow your own tomatoes, you can experiment a bit with varieties that produce lower-acid fruits. Many of the low-acid varieties are quite tasty, have good yields, and the plants are disease-resistant. IC patients across the country have had success in growing low-acid tomato varieties at home. Tomatoes are so popular and seeds so universally available, that you should have no trouble in locating low-acid varieties that will grow well in your area. Of course, even if the crop fails or all the produce turns out to be too acid for your bladder, you are still ahead of the game. Gardening has given you fresh air and exercise, and you can present your friends and family with delectable, home-grown, fresh tomatoes to enjoy.

Low-acid tomato varieties

Several low-acid tomato varieties are listed below, but because growing conditions vary from place to place, not all the ones on the list may be suitable for your area. If you cannot find any of those varieties, some diligent investigation at local libraries, colleges, nurseries, and university cooperative extension offices may turn up the names of other low-acid varieties that will grow where you live. Remember though, that acidity is relative and even low-acid tomatoes are still high enough in acid to bother some people.

I've grown Ace 55, Jet Star, Yellow Pear and others with good results. In general, I've found the yellow or white varieties to be milder in flavor than the red ones, even the low-acid red ones. Because tomatoes have less acidity than some other food items we avoid, you may have an easier time using an antacid preparation to counteract their acidity, and this may be especially true if the tomato is a low-acid variety.

Here's a tip from commercial tomato growers that IC patients may be able to use to advantage, too: Watering throughout the fruit-ripening period will affect the amount of water in the fruit, and thus the flavor. Most people want their tomatoes very tasty, not watery. Produce growers therefore water as little as possible in the last few days before harvest to concentrate the flavor. You may want to experiment with giving the tomatoes more water, rather than less, to see if the more "watery" fruit becomes even less acid. I've found that my ripening tomatoes also tend to crack when they are overwatered, causing them to rot and become moldy if not harvested right away, so be sure to keep an eye on them.

In the following list, resistance to disease is indicated by the initials "V" for verticillium, "N" for nematode, "F" for fusarium, and "A"for anthracnose. Tomato plants are either determinate (grow to a certain size and stop, usually at about 3 feet), or indeterminate (continue to grow very large). Carefully consider the space you have available when you choose the variety. My "Yellow Pear" tomato plant nearly took over the garden! Determinate or indeterminate varieties are indicated below as "Det." or "Ind."

WHITE TOMATOES

***Snowball*.** Fruit white when ripe. Suitable for warm summer regions. According to some authorities, "white" varieties may have lowest acidity of all.

New Snowball. Same as Snowball.

White Beauty. Very low acidity, open-pollinated plant, sweet fruit is creamy white inside and out when ripe. Ind.

YELLOW AND GOLDEN TOMATOES

Golden Boy. Fruit golden yellow, large and firm when ripe. Suitable for Western gardens. Ind., A.

Jubilee. Fruit medium-size and golden orange when ripe. Has some crack resistance, Ind., A.

Jet Star. Widely adapted. Well suited for home growing, very popular in the Northeast. Good yields, Ind., V, F.

Lemon Boy. Fruit bright lemon-yellow when ripe. Well-adapted for the Northeast. Ind., V, F, N, A.

Yellow Pear. Fruit is yellow, pear-shaped and small (about 1" to 1-1/2"). Vigorous growth, good for Midwestern gardens. Ind., A.

PINK AND RED TOMATOES

Ace 55. Fruit red when ripe, late-season producer. Widely adapted where summers are warm. Especially good for Western states. Det., V, F.

Pink Ponderosa. Widely adapted where summers are warm. Large fruit, pink when ripe. Ind.

Spring Giant. Fruit red when ripe, meaty, large. Among milder and less acid of the popular, red, large-fruit varieties. Widely adapted and suitable for areas with cool summers. High yield. Det., V, F.

Sources of tomato seeds and plants

If you can't find low-acid tomato plants or seed locally, here's a seed supplier who stocks most of the low-acid varieties listed, along with hundreds of others. Packets of 100 seeds usually run about $1.50 each, but they have discount prices for large orders. For a catalog, write to: *Tomato Growers Supply Company, P.O. Box 2237, Fort Myers, FL 33902.*

There is also a lady in California who sells low-acid tomato plants and will ship them anywhere in the U.S. All of Lore's plants are the old-fashioned, open-pollinated varieties as opposed to hybrids. She encourages people to save the seeds and plant them again next year. (You can't grow a hybrid by just collecting seeds from the tomatoes this year and planting them next year. You may get second generation plants that are not at all like the parent— if the seeds germinate at all).

She offers twenty-three "heirloom" varieties and says the best bets for low-acidity among her offerings are, *White Beauty*, *Evergreen* (a greenish-gold when ripe), and among the reds, *Costello Genovese.* Plants are $3.50 each, plus handling and shipping charges, (and tax for California residents). These plants, although expensive, can supply you with seeds year after year. If you plant several varieties in your garden, they won't easily cross-pollinate, Lore says. For more information, call or write: *Lore's Best Basil and Herb Farm, P.O. Box 3485, Camarillo, CA 93010; phone, (800) 404-8662.*

Some words of caution

With a bounty of low-acid tomatoes to harvest and enjoy, you may be tempted to can or freeze some for later use. The low-acid tomatoes may require a different canning method than you've used in the past. Appendix B has some information and other resources that will help you decide how to preserve your harvest.

Another interesting fact about tomatoes that you may want to consider comes from the American Academy of Allergy, Asthma and Immunology. They've found that in people who are allergic to tomatoes, the riper the tomato, the more allergenic it becomes. (In terms of acidity, the riper it becomes, the less acid it is).

For some people with IC, acidity main be the main difficulty, whereas others with IC may find that ripeness affects their bladder's reaction more. Everyone's different, so see what works for you. For me, the ones that work best actually seem to be those crunchy, tasteless, horrible "tomatoes" the supermarket sells (and the less luscious looking the better). I've found too, that my sensitivity pattern changes according to the medication I am taking for my IC. Elmiron, for instance, seems to make me more sensitive to acidic foods, but less sensitive to spicy foods.

Monosodium Glutamate (MSG) and Nitrates

MSG

Monosodium glutamate, also known as MSG, is a flavor enhancer and food additive commonly used in prepared and processed foodstuffs. It is also a substance which occurs naturally in some foods. Of all the items on the IC diet, it may be the hardest to avoid and the easiest for newly diagnosed IC patients to identify as a symptom-provoker.

MSG is on the Food and Drug Administration's "Generally Recognized as Safe" (GRAS) list merely because it has been in widespread use for so long. The GRAS rating means it can be used in many food products, but controversy regarding its safety has continued for the last thirty years. (Glutamate is a neurotransmitter which is normally involved in learning and memory, but under certain circumstances can damage or destroy nerve cells by over-stimulating them. It has been shown to affect the nerves through the function of nitric oxide, a substance of interest in the symptomology of IC). In a few scientific studies, a number of chronic conditions and diseases, including Alzheimer's, have recently been linked to glutamate. Although nothing conclusive has been demonstrated in humans, speculation continues and the Alzheimer's Association is following the ongoing research with great interest.

Of more immediate concern to IC patients, particularly those with allergies, is MSG's action as an effective mast cell degranulator. (Degranulation is a term scientists use to refer to the way the cells release histamine and other inflammation-causing substances.) MSG can in fact, provoke symptoms anywhere mast cells are found, including the sinuses and the skin. According to the American Academy of Allergy, Asthma, and Immunology, many people suffer allergic skin reactions to monosodium glutamate, and in others it can trigger asthma attacks.

MSG has also been shown to stimulate nerve cells via the action of nitric oxide, a substance currently under investigation for its involvement in IC. It has also been postulated that the nerve endings in IC bladders are unusually sensitive. Because recent studies have implicated both mast cells and nitric oxide in the pain process of both interstitial cystitis and irritable bowel syndrome, we should approach MSG-containing foods with great caution.

The substance is notorious for causing "Chinese Restaurant Syndrome", an allergic reaction to the MSG which is frequently found in Chinese food. People may experience light-headedness, skin rashes, or difficulty breathing. For centuries, MSG has been favored by Chinese cooks for enhancing the flavor of various dishes. Today though, some Chinese restaurants recognize that their customers may have difficulty with the substance, so they don't use it. Whenever I visit a Chinese restaurant for the first time, I always ask if they use MSG.

Monosodium glutamate used to be made from wheat gluten, but the food additive used today is synthetically manufactured from other materials. Although regarded as safe for human consumption, the FDA does set limits on how much synthetic MSG manufacturers can put in their products. That is no comfort to the many people whose sensitive IC bladders detect even minute amounts.

There are three ways MSG can come to be found in foods. It can be put in processed or packaged food as an intentional additive, it can occur as an unintentional by-product of the food's processing, or it can be there because it is a naturally occurring substance in certain plant products. As an intentional additive, monosodium glutamate is frequently found in sausages and lunch meats, canned soups and bouillon, frozen prepared foods, mayonnaise, sauces, canned crab meat, snack foods, and salad dressings. In these cases it is identified on the label, so one can easily avoid it.

It is more difficult to avoid the MSG which is produced as a by-product of processing or fermentation, because in these cases it won't appear on the food label. MSG can be created when the sodium used in processing combines with the food's natural glutamic acid. Hydrolyzed vegetable protein (HVP), texturized vegetable protein (TVP), autolyzed yeast (often called "yeast extract"), sodium caseinate, and calcium caseinate all contain some MSG.

MSG is created in some fermentation processes too, so that soy sauce, tamari, and miso all contain monosodium glutamate. (Perhaps this is the reason some IC patients are able to use small amounts of certain low-sodium soy sauce brands; they may have less MSG). Aged cheeses also have a form of glutamate. The levels in these fermented, aged, or processed foods are frequently lower than when it has been put into the food as an intentional additive. Nonetheless, even these lower levels may provoke IC bladders.

Foods such as peas, which contain low levels of naturally-occurring glutamate, are the least offensive as far as IC bladders are concerned. Most people with IC can eat peas and the like with no bladder problems. Those who have vulvodynia as well as IC may react to foods such as peas. (In this case, the role of glutamate is unclear and the offending substance may be oxalates. See section on vulvodynia, page 20).

Be wary of products with labels that list "natural flavors," "natural flavoring," or similar terms. Current FDA regulations only require manufacturers to list MSG on the label when the end-product manufacturer intentionally adds it, in its crystalline form. Food labeling regulations are complex and ever-changing. (In past years for instance, soups have been required to list MSG on the label, while mayonnaise products have not.)

Here's another way a fair amount of MSG can get into foods without it being listed specifically on the label: A manufacturer of barbecue sauce, for instance, uses soy sauce and a few spices in the recipe. The soy sauce, by its very nature, may contain a significant amount of MSG. He may also use a tomato paste, ordered from another supplier, which contains added MSG (the barbecue sauce manufacturer is not responsible for listing on *his* label, what the supplier had added to the tomato paste). The maker of the barbecue sauce may also add sodium caseinate, which also contains some MSG, to thicken the sauce. On the label of his barbecue sauce, our hypothetical manufacturer can legitimately list "tomato paste, natural flavoring and spices, sodium caseinate." He hasn't added any crystalline MSG, yet the end product may have enough MSG to set off reactions in people who are sensitive to it.

Nitrates

Nitrates (and their chemical relatives, nitrites) have been added to processed and smoked meat products for many years. And for just as many years they have been triggering pain in IC bladders. Recent research has finally given us a little insight into how and why this may occur.

When you eat a food containing nitrates (or related compounds), they can be metabolized by the body to form nitric oxide (NO). Nitric oxide is a substance involved in many processes in the body. One of the significant things it does, as far as IC is concerned, is that it works with nerves and the circulatory system.

Dr. Shannon Smith and her co-workers at Yale, made news in the IC research community when they discovered that people with IC have less of a nitric oxide-producing enzyme in their urine than healthy people. They figured that this may result in abnormal production and utilization of nitric oxide, and that this abnormality in turn, may trigger IC bladder pain and urgency.

The subject of nitric oxide function is very complex. In large amounts for instance, it can trigger inflammation in muscle tissue, but in small amounts it can keep the muscle relaxed and blood flowing smoothly. It has to be balanced and regulated carefully by the body's own mechanisms. Doctors have suggested that where nitric oxide production is not regulated well, symptoms may result. These symptoms could include: spasms due to lack of blood circulation, inflammation, swelling of tissues due to fluid accumulation, and/or painful chronic stimulation of sensory nerves (which may become overly sensitive).

Because nitric oxide is manufactured and works in such complicated ways in the body, we can't simply dose ourselves with substances that make nitric oxide and solve the problem. We also can't totally avoid substances that make nitric oxide in the body and expect to solve the problem either. Herein rests one of the more curious paradoxes of IC. Nitrates in food (which can form nitric oxide in the body) cause bladder pain, whereas L-arginine (which is also utilized in the production of nitric oxide) has been shown to reduce IC bladder pain.

Until scientists uncover more information about nitric oxide's involvement in IC, we may not know why these things happen. But as patients, we can help ourselves in the meanwhile by taking a few practical steps to reduce our pain and urgency. Avoiding nitrates and nitrites in food has helped many people. And while the long-term consequences of taking L-arginine dietary supplements is not known, some IC patients have favorable results from taking such supplements or increasing their dietary intake of arginine. It is a good subject for discussion with your doctor.

Onions

Some of us with IC have symptom flares when we eat onions, while others don't. Onions are a food for which each person has to find his or her own limits. If you are new to following an IC diet, you will probably find keeping a food diary is helpful when sorting out your individual food reactions. As you test out various items, be sure to write down *all* the ingredients of those which are packaged, canned or bottled. It may be tedious, but it will keep you from jumping to conclusions and giving an innocent food a bad rap. I remember one time I ate some canned French Onion Soup for dinner and felt horrible the next morning, so I naturally assumed that I couldn't tolerate cooked onions. Weeks later I had some homemade onion soup with no problem. I was then perplexed. How could I react one time and not another? Eventually I found it was an additive in the canned soup, not the cooked onions, that caused the flare.

Chives

Onions are members of the lily family, and there are many species, some purely ornamental. Of the species we use for cooking, chives are by far the mildest. People with IC can usually tolerate a little chives, especially if they are cooked. In most recipes, chives aren't a major ingredient— they're just used for a little color or a subtle flavor. I've found, though, that my bladder tolerates raw chives much better than raw green onions, so I use them in some favorite recipes which call for chopped, raw green onions. Substituting chives diminishes the onion-y flavor, but in some recipes that's okay. You might try experimenting to see if that kind of substitution helps you, too.

Chives are often sold as a freeze-dried product in the spice aisle of supermarkets. The dried product is very convenient, but if you substitute it for fresh chives in a recipe, remember to use more. I recall one person with IC telling me that her bladder is so sensitive that dried chives are the only form of onion she can tolerate. She uses them exclusively and liberally, even sprinkling them on salads to give them a little zest.

Chives are very hardy as a house plant and easily grown in a small pot on a sunny window sill. Growing them this way makes the fresh chives always available for use. Just snip as much of the tops as you need. With proper water and a bit of fertilizer, they regrow quickly. If you plant some in your garden, they will grow even faster. Remember that they need quite a bit of nitrogen in the fertilizer. (All members of the onion family are heavy feeders). I have even harvested chives from my garden and dried them for later use. (See instructions for drying herbs at home, in the Miscellaneous section, page 189).

Green onions

Green onions are also okay with many IC patients as long as they are cooked or there is not too much of them in the food. I find the green tops to be milder and more colorful than the bulb onions, so I sometimes substitute green onions for bulb onions in recipes where cooked onions are called for.

My family has some favorite recipes that call for a bit of raw, chopped green onion. On my "good days" I don't have a problem with the raw green onions, so I may just go ahead and use them. On "bad days" though, I'll play it safe and use chives instead in those same recipes, or just make some other food. Green onion tops, like chives, can also be dried for later use.

Shallots (Echalotes)

Shallots are a species of onion with a complex but more intense flavor than the large-bulbed slicing onions. They form a small, brown bulb, often about two inches or less across. You can find them at specialty markets or sometimes in supermarkets. Shallots are a favorite of chefs at many top restaurants, considered essential for French cooking, and can be quite expensive. Cooked, I have found them quite safe, delicious, and a bit different in flavor; but raw, they have the same effect on my bladder as their larger-bulbed relatives— ouch!

If you want to try some of these gourmet onions and can't find them at a market, you can write to the Gourmet Gardener at the address below. They will send you their catalog of gourmet herbs and vegetables. They supply many professional chefs and amateur gourmet cooks. In addition, they have a very interesting list of books on growing and cooking herbs, and some unique kitchen products. (One interesting item is a small muslin bag filled with lavender. Thrown in the dryer with clothes, it gives them a fresh, sweet scent without using any skin-irritating chemicals). Write for a catalog to: *The Gourmet Gardener, 8650 College Blvd., Overland Park, KS 66210-1806.*

Bulb (globe) onions

Most people with IC seem to have trouble with those big, strong, bulb onions that are often sliced and eaten raw, on a hamburger, perhaps. (How I miss being able to eat a slice of sweet red onion!) Yet those of us who wouldn't think of eating a raw slice of onion, may have no trouble with the same slice if it is cooked well. No one knows exactly why IC patients have less trouble with cooked onions. According to the Nutrient Data Laboratory of the USDA, a raw onion and a boiled onion have about the same levels of tryptophan, tyrosine, histamine, and phenylalanine. Onions are not high in tyramine either. It is curious too, that onions grown in low-sulfur soils are reported to be less painful for a few IC sufferers. Perhaps the heat of cooking destroys some sulfur-containing acids. Maybe someday we will know more.

There are two kinds of bulb onions you can buy at the supermarket, sweet onions and storage onions. Most consumers don't know the difference, because they look the same in a big bin at the store. But your bladder might know the difference.

Spring onions or summer onions (referred to by producers as sweet onions) come onto the market around the beginning of April. They have a high sugar content and are generally milder. Storage onions, which are more pungent and have a lower water and sugar content, are the ones you get during the winter months. You may find you are more sensitive to the storage onions than the spring onions, and if so, you may want to be especially attentive to avoiding raw onions in the winter.

Here's another idea which works for at least one person, and may work for you. If your onions are very strong, you might try soaking them in milk. For a slice of onion on a hamburger, for instance, cut the onion in a thin slice. Place in a bowl and cover with milk for an hour or so. Drain the milk and rinse the onion slice carefully before using. Mary, who takes Elmiron and now says her IC only bothers her when she eats food she shouldn't, says this technique has helped her to be able to eat small amounts of raw onions.

Some people say that Vidalia onions are more easily tolerated by their bladders than regular yellow or white slicing onions. The Vidalia onions are grown from the same onion seed as many other onions, but are grown in a low-sulfur soil which naturally occurs in the area around Vidalia, Georgia. As a result of the unique growing conditions, they are much milder and sweeter. They are also hard to get, not always in season, and quite expensive. If you live in the South, you may be able to get them during their season, May through June.

There are a few onion varieties which are milder than the common onions you get in stores, but they can be pricey. A sweet onion that reputedly has 50% more sugar than Vidalias, is the Oso Sweet Onion from South America. I haven't tried this particular onion, but food experts and gourmet food magazines hail it as extremely sweet and mild. It is also expensive and usually available only in specialty stores, January through March. Next to the Vidalias and Osos in sweetness are the Maui onions. They are white to pale yellow and available April through July. I am not sure of their national availability, but they are popular with chefs on the West Coast because of their mild taste.

And here is a tip for keeping raw onions from making your eyes water. It's not your eyes that are irritated so much by the fumes from cut raw onions, as it is your sinuses. (I have found that I am much more sensitive to onion fumes too, since I've had fibromyalgia). Some books say to put on goggles to prevent teary eyes from cut onions, but I've tried that and it didn't work. Here's what I've found does work: putting a swimmer's clip or a weakly sprung clothespin on your nose to keep from breathing through it. It looks silly, but really works! My grandmother had another way: refrigerate the onion. She found chilled onions didn't bother her as much when she cut them.

If all the strategies mentioned fail, and you can't tolerate any member of the onion family (even cooked), consider being tested for food allergies. Some sources have reported onions to be allergenic. If you have a true allergy to onions, chances are it is to a protein in the onion. In that case, cooking it or even reducing the amount of cooked onion in recipes, won't make a significant difference.

Citrus Fruits

Oranges, grapefruit, tangerines, and especially lemons and limes, are big taboos on an IC diet. Their biggest fault IC-wise, is their tangy acidity (although oranges do have a small amount of tyramine). However, a few citrus-loving IC patients have gone to great lengths just to be able to enjoy their favorite fruit now and then. They've come up with some good citrus strategies worth mentioning.

Before exploring what's new or novel, don't forget to try the old tried-and-true standbys to buffer acidity: Tums (calcium carbonate) or a little baking soda in water taken with or after meals.

Here's a new wrinkle on the old acid-buffer technique. Try this and see if it works for you. One longtime IC sufferer says that she uses citrus juices in some recipes without difficulty. The trick, she says, is to use it only in baked recipes that have baking soda or baking powder, and if milk is also added, that's even better. The idea is that the baking soda will neutralize the acid, and in doing so release gas that helps the baked product rise. (This is just like taking a Tums with the food, only it's *in* the food before you eat it). I've tried this, but a little un-neutralized acid must still be left over, because unless I take a Tums, I'm still bothered a bit by it. Nonetheless, I can say that baking with orange juice is less painful, and easier to neutralize with a Tums, than having the same amount in salad dressing.

Some recipes can be altered to include citrus extract or citrus peel as a flavoring, rather than lemon juice. But here's a word of warning about tinkering with recipes for baked goods: you can't just eliminate the citrus juice and expect the same great results. Often baked products depend on an exact balance of acid and alkaline ingredients to initiate a chemical reaction, making them rise.

Oranges

There are two classes of oranges, juicing oranges (like the Valencia variety), and eating oranges (which are usually referred to as "navel" oranges in the supermarket). On the whole, navel oranges are sweeter and less acidic. Because of the difference in acidity, you may find baking soda can more easily avert a flare from eating an orange, than from drinking orange juice.

New on the market are reduced-acid orange juices. One brand, which is available in many localities, is Minute Maid Reduced-Acid frozen concentrate. The reduced-acid orange juice has allowed some IC patients to have orange juice again for the first time in years. If you don't see it at your market, try asking the store manager to stock it.

Lemons

Some lucky people can get away with the small amounts of lemon juice that lend flavor to salad dressings, sauces, and desserts. If this describes you, then Meyer lemons may be a good lemon to experiment with. Meyer lemons, though still tart, are less acidic than popular commercially-grown lemon varieties like Eureka. Meyers are the citrus darling of fine chefs everywhere. Lindsey Shere, pastry chef at Chez Panisse restaurant in Berkeley, California says she likes the really wonderful, very flowery taste and says the complex flavor makes them ideal for desserts. Many professional chefs echo those sentiments.

Thin-skinned Meyer lemons make a great lemon meringue pie with milder flavor and less of the acid "bite" typical of other lemons. The Meyer variety, rumored to actually be a cross between a lemon and an orange, is very suitable for home gardens too, if you'd like to grow your own. The trees are frequently grafted to dwarf stock. I had a very prolific one that had been grafted to dwarf rootstock and was only about 5 feet high and 5 feet across when it was 20 years old, yet it produced dozens of lemons every season (November through March). Even if lemon juice and pulp are not for you, growing them for the pungent peel may be worthwhile. The dried peel is excellent for potpourri and sachets, too. If you've never tried one and would like to, California Citrus Specialties (209-781-0886) sell Meyer lemons by mail-order. (As of this writing, you can get three pounds for about ten dollars, plus shipping). If your area is suitable for growing citrus, and Meyer lemon trees are not locally available, you can mail-order the trees. Here are two suppliers: Just Fruits, Route 2, Box 4818, Crawfordville, FL 32327 (their catalog is $3), and Exotica Rare Fruit Nursery, Box 160 Vista, CA 92083 (phone: 619-724-9093, catalog $2).

Grapefruit

A very acidic fruit— the mere mention of grapefruit sends shivers down the spine of many IC sufferers. Yet some people with very mild cases of IC, or whose IC symptoms are well controlled by medication, do seem to be able to tolerate grapefruit on a limited basis. One lady I know began taking Elmiron when it was in clinical trials. She's been taking it for several years now and the medication has enabled her to once again relish a grapefruit half with breakfast.

There are two new grapefruit tree varieties which have milder-tasting fruit than the older, commercially produced varieties. If you can have grapefruit occasionally, these milder hybrids may let you have more of it, or have it more often. The new hybrids are not true grapefruits, but a cross between a grapefruit and a pummelo. They are so tasty and popular that some commercial growers are beginning to plant them and soon you may be seeing them in supermarkets. These grapefruit-pummelo hybrids are not only relatively less acid, they ripen 3 to 6 months before the true grapefruits. (If you are able to eat these and would like to grow your own, these two lower-acid hybrids are both available grafted to dwarf stock: "Mellow Gold" and "Oro Blanco"). A word of warning: grapefruit and grapefruit juice can both interact in a very dangerous way with some prescription medications. If you are taking medications, be sure to consult your doctor about eating any amount of grapefruit.

Citric acid and citrate additives

A couple of people with IC have posted messages on internet IC newsgroups and bulletin boards about citric acid in over-the-counter medicines or herbal preparations. Read labels carefully because citric acid is added by manufacturers of many items.

Lower-Acid Varieties of High-Acid Fruits

Just as there are lower-acid varieties of tomatoes and citrus, there are also lower-acid varieties of other fruits. Of course, not everyone can tolerate these fruits, even if they are the lower-acid varieties. But if you are one of the fortunate few with a mild case of IC, or you have your symptoms fairly under control, perhaps you can occasionally partake in what is forbidden fruit to many of us.

A word of warning: the fruit varieties listed below are all still very acid— much more so than blueberries and pears. Always remember to let your body be your guide, and if yours is a more severe case of IC or you are extremely sensitive to any amount of these fruits listed below, then it's no doubt best to forego them altogether.

Peaches

There's nothing like sweet peaches. Here are two of the milder, slightly less acid varieties that will grow in many areas of Texas, Florida, California, and the South: "Champagne", a white-fleshed fruit, and "El Dolce" which produces very large, sweet fruit.

You may be able to find these varieties in specialty markets or farmer's markets. For lowest acidity, remember to pick the fruit when it is fully dead-ripe, and the fruit acids have been allowed to convert to sugars as much as possible.

Pineapple Guava

This is a tropical fruit tree that gets twenty feet tall and easily grows in the mild coastal climates of Southern California, the Gulf Coast of Texas and in Florida. (It is a completely different genus and species from the guava.) The fruit is egg-shaped, with an edible pulp and tiny seeds (avoid the skin which is tough and very tart). It tastes like a mix of pineapple and banana. Though this is an acid fruit, the variety "Coolidge" is somewhat milder than other varieties commonly grown.

Loquat

This fruit is very popular in Asia, Central America, and the Mediterranean. The fruit is orange colored, about one to three inches across, and contains one to five seeds. It

This fruit is very popular in Asia, Central America, and the Mediterranean. The fruit is orange colored, about one to three inches across, and contains one to five seeds. It is grown in milder climate areas of the United States, where the subtropical tree grows to twenty-five feet high. Two varieties of this fairly acidic fruit are milder: "Advance" and "Champagne."

Other unusual fruits

You might also be tempted to try some of the more offbeat fruit offerings at specialty markets. Many are very tasty, and if peaches don't bother you, you might find that your bladder can tolerate small amounts of some of them. I haven't seen anyone evaluate these tropical fruits for people with interstitial cystitis, but here are a few that I've personally found to be very acid, so beware: kiwi, papaya, tangelo, kumquat, guava, mountain papayas, and starfruit.

PART TWO

KEY TO THE RECIPE SYMBOLS

I've included some helpful symbols next to each recipe name, you so can immediately identify those recipes that may interest you most. Also, if you are looking for a comprehensive listing of a certain kind of recipe, check the two special indexes in Appendix E: the Vegetarian Index and the Low-Oxalate Index.

Some recipes are only "IC-safe" if a canned, bottled, or packaged ingredient is "safe". (For example, a soup that uses canned chicken broth as a base can be "safe" if the chicken broth is MSG-free. Many brands of canned chicken broth contain MSG, but a few don't.) I've listed some "IC-safe" brands and products in Appendix B, but you may have found other favorites. To assist in finding the brands I've listed, or substitutes, Appendix B also has a list of specialty stores where you are likely to find these products.

Symbol	*Meaning*
★	Rather than calling for a specific "IC-safe" brands in each recipe, I've placed a symbol next to ingredients likely to "make or break" the recipe in terms of causing symptom flares. This symbol alerts you that a "safe" brand or an alternative product is listed on pages 205 through 207 in Appendix B, The IC Pantry.
✿	Denotes a recipe that does not use meat or fish, but may use eggs or dairy products. Also denotes recipes that have variations suitable for vegetarians.
✓	Denotes a recipe that combines features of an IC diet and a low-oxalate diet, or has a variation that is suitable for a low-oxalate diet. (See following page for a listing of the omitted high-oxalate foods).

For the convenience of women with both IC and vulvodynia, who are juggling the requirements of a low-oxalate diet *and* an IC diet, recipes displaying the ✓ symbol also

For the convenience of women with both IC and vulvodynia, who are juggling the the requirements of a low-oxalate diet *and* an IC diet, recipes displaying the ✓ symbol also omit the high-oxalate foods listed below. Please note this is not a comprehensive list of all foods containing significant levels of oxalates, but rather a list of those which I believe to be the worst offenders according to women diagnosed with vulvodynia. Women with more severe cases may wish to omit some additional foods, and may also find *The Low-Oxalate Cookbook* (Vulvar Pain Foundation, 1997) helpful. See Appendix D for more information on the Vulvar Pain Foundation (VPF).

beets
beans of all kinds
blueberries
blackberries
black pepper (in large amounts)
celery
chard
citrus peel
collards
dandelion greens
dried figs
eggplant
escarole
garbanzo beans
green bell peppers
grits
hominy
kale
leeks
mustard greens
okra
parsley
parsnips
rutabaga
sardines
sesame seeds
spelt
spinach
summer squash, yellow
sweet potatoes
turnip greens
watercress
wheat bran
wheat germ
whole wheat products
yams

Portion sizes and calories

With the exception of a few, most recipes in this book serve two to four people. Also, for the convenience of those who are watching their weight, cookies, cakes, pies, and other dessert-type recipes have a per-serving calorie count. (Caloric information is based on data from the U.S. Dept. of Agriculture's Nutrient Data Laboratory).

APPETIZERS

Asparagus Roll Appetizers ✿✓

makes 12

12 asparagus spears, cooked
½ tsp. garlic powder
1 tsp. olive oil
3 Tbsp. margarine, softened
6 slices fresh white bread

Blend garlic powder and olive oil into the margarine. Cut slices of bread in half (making two rectangles), and trim crusts. Spread each piece of bread with seasoned margarine. Trim asparagus spears so that each is about a half-inch longer than the bread is wide. Place a spear on each slice of bread and roll up, secure with fancy toothpick, or tie in a bundle with fresh chives.

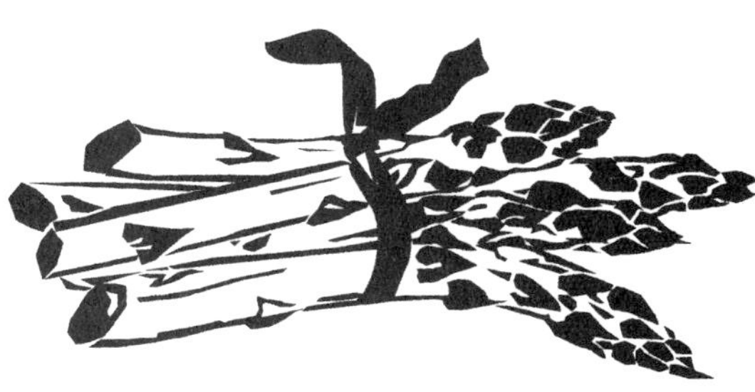

Mini-Corn with Herb Butter ✿✓

makes 12

Everyone will enjoy these zesty little corn-on-the-cobs at summer parties.

3 medium-sized ears of corn, trimmed and shucked
6 Tbsp. margarine or butter
2 cloves garlic, minced
¾ tsp. onion salt
¼ tsp. dried basil
pinch dried marjoram

Bring a large pot of water to a boil. Cut each ear of corn in sections about 1 to 1½ inches thick. Drop corn in water and let cook about six or seven minutes. Remove and drain.

Meanwhile, melt butter in a small pan over medium heat and cook garlic until tender. Add onion salt and remove from heat.

Crumble the basil and marjoram between fingers or crush with a mortar and pestle. Stir the dried basil, dried marjoram into the hot butter.

Drizzle butter over hot corn and serve on a warm platter.

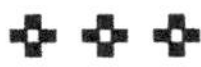

Hard-Boiled... or Raw?

If you forget what's what in the fridge, here's a quick way to tell if that egg is hard-boiled or raw: put the egg on a counter or other flat surface and spin it like a top. A hard-boiled egg will spin smoothly, but a raw one will wobble and quickly come to a stop.

Tarragon Dip ✿

makes 1 cup

1 c. cottage cheese
2 Tbsp. fresh parsley, chopped fine
2 Tbsp. fresh chives, snipped
1 tsp. dried tarragon
¼- ½ tsp. coarse-grind black pepper
crackers ★

Blend cottage cheese with parsley, chives and tarragon. Place on a plate or in a bowl. Sprinkle black pepper over top. Surround with crackers for scoops.

Cucumber variation: Instead of crackers, use thick slices of cucumber for scoops. Wash and scrub the cucumber thoroughly. Cut off ends, then run a fork down the length of the cucumber to peel stripes of skin off.

Slice cucumber in ¼-inch thick slices. After slicing cucumber, submerge slices in ice water for ½ hour. Dry the cucumber slices and arrange around edge of the dip dish.

California Caraway Spread 

makes about 3 cups

8 oz. cream cheese
½ c. milk
1 Tbsp. caraway seed
1 tsp. onion salt
¼ tsp. dried thyme
2½ c. Monterey Jack cheese, grated

With electric mixer, blend cream cheese and milk until smooth. Stir in caraway seed, onion salt, thyme, and Monterey Jack cheese.

Scoop into a serving bowl, cover with plastic wrap, and chill for at least two hours before serving. Serve with crackers or melba toast rounds, and small hors d'oeuvre spreaders.

Caraway dip variation: Add more milk to the chilled spread, beating until smooth and creamy. Radishes, thick slices of bell pepper, or carrot sticks make good scoops.

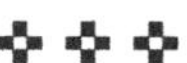

Parsley and Dill Dip

makes 1 cup

2 tsp. beef bouillon base ★
1¼ c. "sour cream" base (see recipe in Miscellaneous section, pg 187)
1 Tbsp. fresh parsley, chopped fine
¼ tsp. garlic powder
¼ tsp. onion salt
½ tsp. dried dill weed
crackers ★

Mix the beef base with a small amount of the "sour cream" base, mashing and blending until thoroughly combined. Blend in the rest of the ingredients. Chill at least one hour before serving. Serve with chilled cooked shrimp, carrots, radishes or celery sticks.

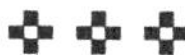

Faux-Boursin Cheese Ball ✿✓

1 8-oz. pkg. cream cheese (softened)
1 tsp. milk
¼ tsp. garlic powder
¾ tsp. dried oregano
½ tsp. dried thyme
¼ tsp. onion salt
¼ tsp. dried basil
¼ tsp. dried marjoram
¼ tsp. black pepper (see variation)
⅛ tsp. dried sage, crumbled
½ c. finely chopped almonds

Blend together the cream cheese, milk, and all the remaining ingredients except the nuts. Mix until smooth. Wrap in plastic wrap or wax paper, making the shape generally that of a ball. Chill about 1¼ hours.

Remove from refrigerator, shape into more of a ball and roll in chopped nuts. Set on serving plate and chill another half hour.

To serve, surround with small spreader knives and crackers, toasted french bread rounds, zucchini slices, or melba toast rounds.

Low-oxalate variation: Same as above, but omit the black pepper.

Clam Dip

makes about 1½ cups

1 8-oz. pkg. cream cheese (softened)
1 7-oz. can minced clams, drained ★
3 Tbsp. clam juice (reserved from clams)
½ c. cottage cheese
2 Tbsp. milk
¼ tsp. allspice
½ tsp. pepper
dash salt

Drain clams and reserve the 3 Tbsp. clam juice. Beat together the cream cheese and clam juice until smooth. Process cottage cheese and milk in a blender or food processor until fairly smooth consistency. Add clams and process a few seconds more. Fold cottage cheese mixture, allspice, garlic powder and pepper into cream cheese. Chill and serve with whole wheat crackers or chilled, cooked, large shrimp.

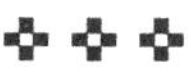

Quick Vegetarian Hors d'Oeuvres

Melon-Nut Crackers ✿✓

Buy salted cashew butter (or purchase unsalted and mix in ½ tsp. salt per ¼ cup cashew butter) and spread it on crackers, making a bit of an indentation in the middle of the nut butter. Add a small dollop of honey in the center, then press a sliver of honeydew melon into the honey and nut butter.

Cashew-Celery Crackers ✿

Mix ¼ cup finely chopped celery and ¼ cup unsalted cashew butter (it helps to microwave the nut butter a few seconds to get it to room temperature if it has been refrigerated). Spread on crackers then top each cracker with 4 or 5 dried currants (or chopped dates or chopped, dried prune bits if desired).

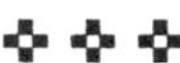

Broiled Cheese Appetizers ✿✓

makes about 12

1 Tbsp. margarine
1 green onion
1 egg white
Muenster cheese, grated
french bread slices

Saute green onion in margarine until soft, remove from pan and set aside to cool 5 minutes. In bowl, beat egg white until frothy. Add Muenster cheese and cooled onion to egg white. Spread on top of french bread slices and broil until bubbly. Watch carefully to avoid scorching. Remove and cool slightly. Cut each piece of french bread in quarters. Serve warm.

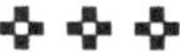

Hot Broccoli-Cheese Tartlets ✿✓

makes about 20

1½ c. small broccoli florets, fresh
1½ c. flour
¼ tsp. salt
¼ c. margarine, softened
3 Tbsp. olive oil
5 Tbsp. cold water

1 egg
1 egg white
1 c. grated Mozzarella cheese
1 Tbsp. fresh chives, chopped
1 mini-muffin pan (2-inch cups)

Cut up broccoli, discarding stems bigger than half an inch across. Cook florets until soft, then drain and set aside. Preheat oven to 400° F.

In a large bowl mix salt and flour. Cut in margarine and olive oil with a pastry blender until like coarse crumbs. Add water and stir until dough forms a ball. Roll out on a floured surface to ⅛ inch thick. Cut circles with a 2½-inch cutter and press into muffin pans.

Beat egg and egg white until frothy and light, about a minute, then stir in grated cheese and chives.

Place a small floret in each pastry cup. Top each with about a teaspoon of the cheese-egg mixture. Bake at 400° F. for about 10 minutes, just until tops start to turn golden brown. Serve warm.

BREAD AND BREAKFAST

Quick Brown Sugar Coffee Cake ✿✓

serves 4 to 6

1 tsp. baking powder
¼ tsp. baking soda
½ tsp. cinnamon
½ tsp. nutmeg
⅛ tsp. cream of tartar
⅛ tsp. coriander

1¼ c. all-purpose flour
¼ tsp. salt
1 c. light brown sugar
⅓ c. margarine or butter

½ c. milk
1 egg

Preheat oven to 375° F. Mix together in a small dish, the baking powder, baking soda, cinnamon, nutmeg, cream of tartar, and coriander. Set aside. In another bowl, mix flour salt, and brown sugar. Cut in the margarine until crumbly. Set aside ¾ cup of crumbs. Mix remaining crumbs with reserved spices.

When mixed well, beat milk and egg into the spiced crumbs just until thoroughly mixed. Pour into a greased and floured 9-inch square cake pan. Sprinkle reserved crumbs on top.

Bake at 375° F. for 25 minutes (or until toothpick in center comes out clean). Serve while still warm. (Make crumbs the night before and refrigerate for a quick morning assembly).

Pumpkin Breakfast Bread ✿✓

makes 1 loaf

This fragrant loaf is irresistible warm from the oven on a cool morning. Measure and mix the dry ingredients together the night before, and making it is a snap.

1⅔ c. all-purpose flour
1 tsp. cinnamon
½ tsp. ginger
½ tsp. nutmeg
½ tsp. allspice
½ tsp. salt
1¼ tsp. baking soda
⅛ tsp. cream of tartar
½ c. margarine, softened
1⅓ c. light brown sugar, packed
2 eggs
1 c. canned or homemade pumpkin puree
⅓ c. lowfat milk
⅓ c. finely chopped cashews

Generously coat a loaf pan with non-stick cooking spray, then dust with flour. Combine first eight ingredients and mix together well. In another bowl, cream together the margarine and brown sugar, then beat in eggs, pumpkin and milk. Beat the liquid into to the dry ingredients, mixing well. Stir in nuts.

Pour into prepared pan and bake at 350° F. for 1 hour. Let cool for ten minutes before removing and slicing. (These loaves freeze well too).

Berry-Filled Coffee Cake ✿

serves 8

An elegant coffee cake, I like serving this to guests while still warm from the oven, on Christmas morning.

For the crumb topping:

2 Tbsp. sugar

6 Tbsp. all-purpose flour

1 Tbsp. margarine, melted

1 Tbsp. margarine (stick kind, refrigerated)

For the berry filling:

1 Tbsp. flour

6 Tbsp. sugar

1½ c. fresh or frozen blueberries (or blackberries)

⅛ tsp. nutmeg

⅛ tsp. baking soda (neutralizes any berry acidity)

1 tsp. water

For the cake:

½ c. margarine, softened

½ c. sugar

1 egg

½ tsp. almond extract

1½ c. all-purpose flour

1¼ tsp. baking powder

½ tsp. baking soda

⅛ tsp. salt

¾ c. milk

Preheat oven to 350° F. and grease and flour a 10-inch tart pan with a removable bottom. Start with crumb topping: Sift together the flour and sugar, cut in the melted margarine and the chunk of refrigerated stick margarine with a pastry cutter. This should give a texture that has both coarse crumbs and fine crumbs. Set aside.

Mix the flour and sugar for the filling in a small saucepan. Add the remaining filling ingredients. Bring to a rolling boil over medium heat while stirring. When done cooking, liquid will be deep reddish purple and thickened, with no foam. Set aside to cool.

Cream margarine and sugar for the cake batter, beating together until light. Beat in egg and extract until fluffy. In another bowl, thoroughly combine the flour, baking powder, baking soda, and salt. Add dry ingredients alternately with milk to the egg mixture while beating. Spread out half the batter in bottom of pan. With a spatula, spread berry filling on top of batter, to within half an inch of outside edge. Spoon out remaining batter on top of filling, in tablespoon-sized globs, spreading slightly. Sprinkle on the crumb topping. Bake for 35 to 40 minutes at 350° F., until top is golden brown. Let cool 15 minutes in pan before removing to a serving plate. Serve warm or cooled.

Pear variation: Use sliced pears instead of berries, and substitute ⅛ tsp. cinnamon for nutmeg in filling. Omit baking soda in filling. In cake, omit almond extract and use 1 tsp. vanilla extract instead.

Currant-Filled Sweet Rolls ✿

makes 8 large rolls

Cinnamon-Oat Bread dough (1 recipe)
½ c. sugar
2 tsp. cinnamon
⅓ c. dried currants

Icing:
1 c. powdered sugar
1 Tbsp. butter, melted
1 tsp. vanilla
milk (or water)

Make Cinnamon-Oat Bread dough according to recipe (pg. 85), letting rise just once and punching down. After punching dough down and kneading 4 or 5 times, let dough rest 10 minutes.

Roll out into a rectangle about 8 inches wide and 15 inches long. Brush dough with water, then sprinkle with mixture of cinnamon and sugar. Sprinkle with currants.

Roll up like a jelly roll, starting at a short side. Seal edge by pressing into the dough. Cut into 8 slices, each about 1 inch thick.

Place slices in a greased 8 x 12-inch baking pan. Cover with damp cloth and let rise till double, about 45 minutes. Bake at 375° F. for 20 minutes. Remove from pan to cool.

To make icing:

Add melted butter and vanilla to sugar in a small bowl, blending with spoon or spatula. Add milk slowly, a teaspoon at a time, blending until spreading consistency. Spread on cooled or slightly warm rolls before serving.

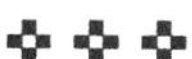

Clover Honey Bread 

A perfect quickbread for leisurely Saturday morning breakfasts, the sweet, floral taste of clover comes through in every tender crumb.

½ c. chopped dates ★
½ c. warm water
½ c. margarine or butter, softened
⅔ c. sugar
¼ c. clover honey
⅓ c. "sour cream" base (see recipe, in Miscellaneous, pg. 187)
2 eggs
1 tsp. vanilla extract
½ c. finely chopped almonds
2 tsp. grated lemon peel (optional, see note)
1½ c. all-purpose flour
2 tsp. baking powder
¼ c. milk

In a small bowl, combine water and dates and set aside for 5 minutes. Preheat oven to 325° F. Meanwhile, beat together the margarine and sugar until fluffy. Add honey, "sour cream" base, eggs, and vanilla, beating just until blended. Drain the dates.

Stir almonds, grated peel, dates into the batter. Sift together flour and baking powder. Alternately add the dry ingredients and the milk to the batter while stirring.

Turn into a greased and floured 9 x 5 x 3-inch loaf pan, then bake at 325° F. for 1 hour and 5 minutes. Let cool 10 minutes before removing from the pan.

Note: For a lower oxalate version, you can substitute ½ tsp. lemon extract for the lemon peel, or eliminate the lemon altogether and increase the vanilla to 1½ tsp.

Holiday variation: If the coloring or preservatives in candied fruit sold during the holidays doesn't bother your bladder, you can add 2 Tbsp. each of chopped green and red candied cherries to the batter. Decrease sugar by 3 Tbsp.

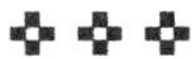

Featherlight Pancakes ✿✓

makes about 10, 6-inch pancakes

1 c. plus 2 Tbsp. all-purpose flour
4 tsp. cream of tartar
2 tsp. baking soda
½ tsp. salt

2 beaten eggs
1 c. milk
3 tsp. salad oil

Combine dry ingredients and mix very well. In a separate small bowl, whisk eggs. Blend in milk and oil. Have skillet or griddle warmed up, because the batter has to be used quickly once it's made. (Griddle is at the right temperature for cooking pancakes when a drop of water dances).

Pour milk mixture into dry ingredients and blend with a spoon just until thoroughly moistened. (Batter will still have a few small lumps). Pour or spoon out in 6-inch circles, turning over when top starts to dry and bubbles begin to set.

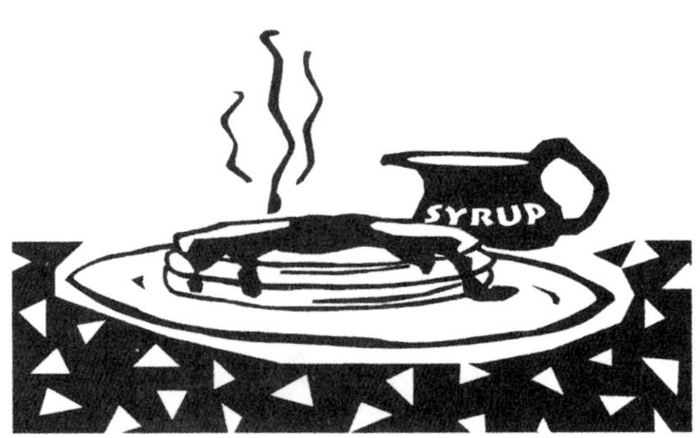

Butter and Blueberry Pancake Topping ✿

serves 3

4 Tbsp. butter or margarine
½ c. sugar
1 c. fresh blueberries
dash nutmeg

Melt butter in saucepan and add sugar mixing well. Cook over medium heat, stirring constantly, until it boils and turns syrupy and thick. Add blueberries and nutmeg. Continue cooking and stirring until blueberries are cooked through and mixture boils again, about 2 minutes. Remove from heat and cool slightly before serving over waffles, pancakes, or french toast.

Ice Cream for Breakfast?

If you've ever inadvertently left some ice cream out and it melted, you know that refreezing it doesn't work— yuck! Next time, just refrigerate it and use it for breakfast. Add it to hot cooked oatmeal, or use it in place of the milk in waffles or pancakes. If you pour it over dry, granola-type cereal, your kids will love it!

Pears in Cinnamon Syrup ✿✓

serves 4

½ c. butter
1 c. sugar
2 pears (not overripe), peeled, chopped
¼ tsp. cinnamon
warm waffles

Melt butter in saucepan and add sugar. mixing well. Cook over medium heat, stirring constantly, until sugar turns syrupy and thick, and begins to brown. As soon as it begins to turn brown, add the chopped pears and cinnamon. Continue cooking and stirring until pears are cooked through.

Remove from heat and cool slightly before serving over waffles. (It's also good on pancakes, or as a dessert sauce over pound cake or ice cream.)

Oatmeal Waffles ✿✓

makes 2, 10-inch waffles

¼ c. quick-cooking oatmeal
1½ c. all-purpose flour
3 tsp. baking powder
¼ tsp. salt
1¾ c. low fat milk
1 egg yolk
⅓ cup salad oil
3 egg whites

In food processor or chopper, chop oatmeal until texture is like that of cornmeal. Mix together the oatmeal, flour, baking powder, and salt. Whisk the milk, egg yolk and oil into the dry ingredients, stirring after each addition.

Preheat the waffle iron. (When a drop of water dances and sizzles, it's ready to use).

In a separate bowl, beat egg whites until soft peaks form. Gently fold egg whites into the batter. Bake in a heated waffle iron.

Nut waffles: Sprinkle 2 Tbsp. finely chopped almonds, cashews, (or, pecans if you can tolerate them) on top before baking.

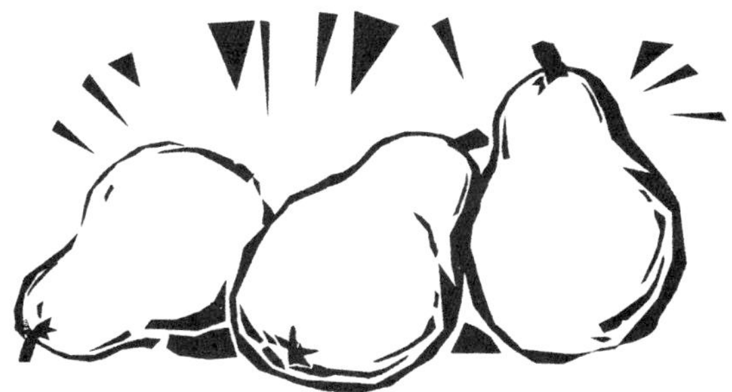

French Toast with a New Twist

Here are two recipes that give the old breakfast standby a novel and decidedly healthier twist. The first version replaces the syrup or jelly topping with fiber- and vitamin-packed fruit and nuts. The second is especially appealing to children— a bladder-friendly version of a fried peanut butter sandwich!

French Toast #1 

serves 2

2 egg whites
⅛ tsp. salt
¼ tsp. cinnamon
⅓ c. milk
4 slices of bread
margarine, or non-stick cooking spray

For pear and nut topping:

2 ripe pears, peeled and sliced
2 tsp. honey
¼ tsp. cinnamon
¼ c. chopped salted cashews

Puree pears in a blender or food processor. In saucepan heat pear puree, honey, and cinnamon until it bubbles. Set aside and keep warm.

Spray skillet with non-stick cooking spray or melt margarine in skillet, being careful not to burn. In a bowl, whisk egg whites, salt, cinnamon, and milk. Dip bread in egg batter, then fry. Pour pear puree over toast, top with nuts.

French Toast #2

serves 2

3 or 4 Tbsp. salted cashew butter
4 slices of whole wheat bread
1 pear
3 Tbsp. margarine or butter
dash mace
1 egg
2 egg whites
⅓ c. milk

Spoon out cashew butter and heat (in microwave, or small saucepan) until warm. If using unsalted nut butter, add a dash of salt.

Spread one side of each of two slices of bread with nut butter. Peel pear and cut off very thin slices (about an eighth of an inch thick) with a paring knife.

In skillet, heat margarine and quickly fry the pear slices about 30 seconds over medium heat. Remove pears and place on top of nut butter. Sprinkle with dash of mace, then top with other slice of bread. Beat egg, egg whites and milk together until frothy and well blended.

Dip the assembled sandwich carefully into the egg mixture, then fry as usual on both sides for french toast.

Note: Almond butter and apricots work well too, if your bladder can tolerate those. And if your bladder can tolerate raisins, they are great with the pears.

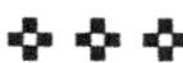

Great Omelets

If your pan isn't absolutely squeaky clean, an omelet can stick. Before you use it for an omelet, pour about a tablespoon of salt in your skillet and rub and polish the surface with a paper towel. The salt will remove any unseen particles that may cause the omelet to stick.

Gingerbread Breakfast Muffins ✿

makes 18

4 c. all purpose flour
2 tsp. baking powder
1 tsp. baking soda
⅔ c. sugar
1 tsp. salt
1 tsp. ginger
1 tsp. cinnamon
½ tsp allspice
1 c. toasted wheat germ

6 eggs
½ c. molasses
1 Tbsp. fresh grated orange peel
⅔ c. salad oil
2 c. milk

In a large bowl mix together very well the flour, baking powder and baking soda. Mix in the rest of the dry ingredients.

In another bowl, whisk the eggs slightly, then whisk in molasses, peel, oil, and milk.

Add liquid mixture all at once to the dry ingredients and stir just until thoroughly moistened. Divide the batter among 18 paper bake cups or greased muffin tins and bake at 375° F. for 25 minutes. Serve warm or cooled.

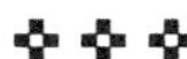

Perfect Blueberry Muffins ✿

makes 12

2 c. flour
⅓ c. sugar
1 tsp. baking powder
½ tsp. baking soda
½ tsp. salt

3 eggs, beaten until frothy
1 c. milk
⅓ c. canola oil
1 tsp. vanilla
¾ cup fresh blueberries

Preheat oven to 400° F. and grease muffin pans, or use paper bake cups. Mix together the first five ingredients in a bowl, making a crater in the center. Set aside. In another bowl, beat egg, then add milk, oil, and vanilla, stirring to blend. Pour the liquid mixture and blueberries all at once into the center of the dry ingredients. Stir quickly, just until dry ingredients are moistened. (If over-beaten, muffins will be tough and have a dull crust). Fill bake cups and bake at 400° F. until golden, about 25 minutes.

If you don't use bake cups, remove muffins from pans while cooling to keep crusts from getting soggy and sticky. (You can use frozen blueberries in this recipe, but do not thaw them before adding).

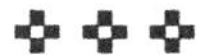

Almond-Date Muffins ✿✓

makes 12

2 c. flour
⅓ c. sugar
1 tsp. baking powder
½ tsp. baking soda
½ tsp. salt

6 egg whites, beaten until frothy
1 c. milk
⅓ c. canola oil
¼ tsp. vanilla
½ tsp. almond extract
½ c. chopped almonds
⅓ c. chopped dates

Preheat oven to 400° F. and grease muffin pans, or use paper bake cups. Mix the dry ingredients in a bowl, making a crater in the center. In another bowl, beat egg. Then add milk, oil, vanilla and almond extract to the eggs, stirring to blend well.

Pour milk mixture, almonds, and dates all at once into the center of the dry ingredients. Stir quickly, just until dry ingredients are moistened. (If over-beaten, muffins may be tough).

Fill twelve standard-sized bake cups and bake at 400° F until golden, about 25 minutes. (If you don't use paper bake cups, remove muffins from pans while cooling to keep crusts from getting soggy and sticky).

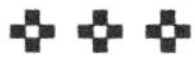

Poppy Seed Whole Wheat Muffins ✿

makes 24 mini-muffins, or 12 regular-size

Poppy seeds add a nutty crunch to this aromatic, citrus-flavored muffin. They are wonderful served with lamb or Middle Eastern vegetable dishes.

1 c. whole wheat flour
1¼ c. all-purpose flour
½ c. sugar
2 Tbsp. poppy seeds
1 Tbsp. baking powder
½ tsp. salt
⅛ tsp. turmeric
1 egg
¾ tsp. vanilla extract
1⅓ c. milk
3 Tbsp. margarine, melted
3 Tbsp. vegetable oil
1 Tbsp. orange peel, freshly grated (or 1½ tsp. orange extract)

Preheat oven to 375° F. and coat the insides of muffin pans with margarine, or use paper baking cups. Thoroughly combine the first seven dry ingredients in a large bowl and set aside.

In another bowl, beat the egg until frothy with an electric mixer, about 30 seconds on medium speed. Add vanilla extract, milk, melted margarine, and oil to the egg then beat again until blended. Stir in orange peel or orange extract.

Make a well in the dry ingredients and add the liquid ingredients. Fold the dry ingredients into the liquid by hand just until mixture is uniform (over-mixing will make the muffins tough). Divide the batter evenly among 12 regular-sized baking cups or 24 mini-muffin cups.

Bake at 375° F. until a toothpick in the center comes out clean, about 20 minutes for mini-muffins, or 25 minutes for regular sized.

Turn out muffins and let cool on a wire rack. These are at their best when served warm.

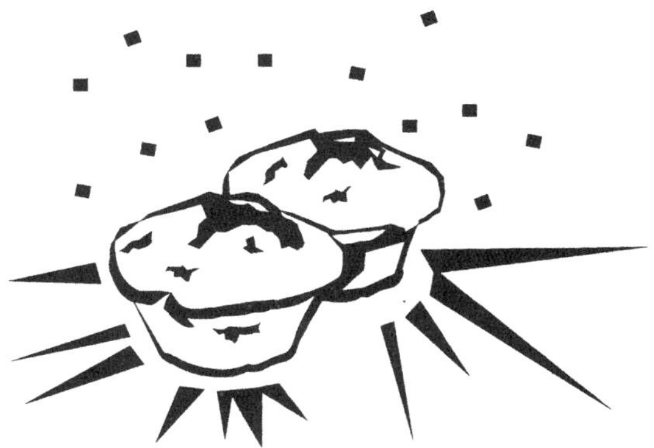

Blueberry Corn Muffins ✿

makes 12

1 c. cornmeal

1 c. all-purpose flour

½ c. sugar

4¼ tsp. baking powder

½ tsp. salt

1 egg

2 egg whites

1 c. plus 2 Tbsp. milk

⅓ c. margarine, melted

¾ c. frozen blueberries

Thoroughly mix together in a large bowl, the cornmeal, flour, sugar, baking powder, and salt. Make a crater in the center of the dry ingredients.

Melt the butter in a small dish or pan. Set the dry ingredients and melted butter aside for the moment. Preheat oven to 400° F.

In another bowl, slightly beat egg and egg whites, then beat in milk. Add melted butter to the milk mixture, then quickly add the liquid ingredients to the dry ingredients. Fold together just until all is moistened. (Over-beating causes tough, heavy muffins).

Gently fold in the *unthawed* blueberries and divide among 12 well-buttered muffin cups. Bake at 400° F. for 30 minutes. Cool slightly before serving.

Note: For an interesting variation, use cornmeal made from blue corn.

Wheat-Allergy and Low-Sodium Baking

Gluten Intolerance or Wheat Allergy

If you have a gluten intolerance you can often replace wheat flour with oat flour, or a combination of oat and rice flour. Neither have gluten.

Oat flour is very good for breading and frying things, and it is also good as a thickening agent. It does, however, look sort of gray and unappealing in sauces. In baked recipes you can substitute one cup of oat flour for each cup of wheat flour with no other changes.

You can also substitute half a cup of oat flour and half a cup of rice flour for a cup of wheat flour in baked goods, but it may be a little dry. (To increase moisture, try adding a bit more oil, some pear juice instead of some of the sugar, or add some pre-soaked dates or currants). The oat/rice flour does make an excellent pie crust, though.

If you have a wheat allergy, you can also replace wheat flour with corn flour in many baked recipes. (If you do, use a little more baking powder than your original recipe calls for because corn flour is heavier).

Baking for a Low-Sodium Diet

Baking soda and baking powder both help baked products rise by creating gas bubbles during baking. Both have loads of sodium in them too, unfortunately, so if your doctor is having you limit your sodium intake, you will probably want to use as little of these leavening agents as possible.

Salt also has sodium, so you will probably be cutting back on that too. Often salt can be drastically reduced or even eliminated from a recipe if it's only there to enhance the flavor. You can't cut back the salt very much in yeast breads though, because it needs to be there to control the growth of the yeast.

If you are thinking of experimenting with your baked goods recipes, or are creating completely new recipes, here are some minimum amounts of salt and baking powder that you should use. Remember, these are only a guide:

For biscuits, muffins, and waffles -
Use 1¼ teaspoons baking powder per cup of flour.

For cakes -
Use 1 teaspoon of baking powder per cup of flour.

For yeast breads -
As a bare minimum, use ¼ teaspoon of salt per cup of flour in yeast breads.

Cinnamon Oatmeal Muffins ✿

makes 12

1 c. lowfat milk

⅔ c. quick-cooking oats

¼ c. wheat germ

1½ c. all purpose flour

⅓ c. sugar

4½ tsp. baking powder

1 tsp cinnamon

½ tsp. salt

2 eggs

2 egg whites

5 Tbsp. melted margarine or butter

Combine oats and milk and set aside. Meanwhile in another bowl, stir together wheat germ, flour, sugar, baking powder, cinnamon and salt. Make a crater in the center of the dry ingredients. Beat together the eggs and egg whites until light-colored and frothy. Melt butter and pour into center of dry ingredients. Quickly add oatmeal and eggs, then stir just until the dry ingredients are moistened. Grease the muffin tins well with butter and divide batter evenly among 12 tins. Bake at 400°F. for 25 minutes.

Note: These are also good with ¼ c. of added raisins, dried currants, or chopped nuts. Add 2 tsp. more milk if you add raisins or currants.

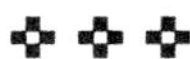

Sage Biscuits 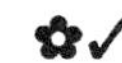

makes about 8

The hint of sage makes these airy biscuits a delightful accompaniment for poultry dishes.

2 c. all-purpose flour
4 tsp. baking powder
1 tsp. dried sage
½ tsp. salt
¼ tsp. baking soda
5 Tbsp. margarine, softened
⅔ c. milk

Preheat oven to 450° F. Combine flour, baking powder, sage, salt, and baking soda. Cut in margarine with a pastry blender until like coarse cornmeal. Add milk all at once, then quickly stir just until uniform consistency. Turn out on floured surface, kneading gently only two or three times.

As soon as dough is not sticky, pat out until dough is about three-quarters of an inch thick. Cut with a 2½-inch round biscuit cutter, and place on an ungreased cookie sheet. Bake biscuits at 450° F. for about 10 to 12 minutes, just until golden brown on top.

Note: For an interesting look, cut these out with a star-shaped cookie cutter. Be sure that your cutter is sharp.

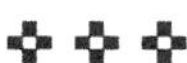

Homestyle Biscuits 

makes 12

2 c. flour
4 tsp. baking powder
½ tsp. salt
4 Tbsp. stick margarine
¾ c. lowfat milk
milk, to brush tops

Mix flour, baking powder and salt together in a large bowl. Melt margarine and pour over dry ingredients. Cut in with a pastry blender until texture is like cornmeal. Add milk and blend just until the dough holds together. Preheat oven to 425° F. Turn dough out on a floured board, dusting it with flour. Knead slightly. When dough is no longer sticky, roll out and cut circles about ¾ of an inch thick. Place biscuits on cookie sheet, edges touching. Brush tops with milk. Bake at 425° F. for 10-12 min.

No More Hockey Pucks

Biscuits should be light and airy with a thin, tender, golden brown crust. Before I learned some tricks of biscuit making, my kids would say, "Mom's making hockey pucks again!" Here's some do's and dont's to keep your biscuits from being as tough and hard as a hockey puck:

1. Before baking, make sure the oven is preheated and at the correct temperature. A hot oven is needed to bake good biscuits.

2. Work quickly, and as lightly as possible, when adding the butter or margarine to the flour. A pastry blender works better than a fork to cut it in. Don't over-work the dough.

3. After adding the liquid and turning out on a floured surface, knead it gently and lightly, as little as possible. Biscuit dough needs less kneading than bread dough, because you don't want to develop the gluten.

4. Don't use a glass or dull object to cut out the biscuits. Use a sharp cookie cutter, a knife, or a biscuit cutter. A dull cutter will squash air pockets out of the biscuits, keeping them from rising.

Buttery Whole Wheat Biscuits ✿

makes 6

⅔ c. white flour

⅓ c. whole wheat flour

2 tsp. baking powder

¼ tsp. salt

2 Tbsp. butter (at room temperature)

6 Tbsp. milk

Thoroughly mix the two flours, baking powder, and salt together. Cut in the butter until mixture has texture of cornmeal. Add milk and blend with a spoon, just until the mixture holds together. Turn out dough on a floured board, dusting dough lightly with white flour. Fold over a couple of times, dusting lightly with flour each time.

When dough is no longer sticky, roll out and cut 2½-inch circles about ¾ inch thick. Arrange on a cookie sheet so that the edges touch, and bake in a 425° F. oven until tops are golden, about 10-15 minutes.

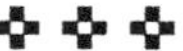

Chive Drop Biscuits 

makes about 8

1 c. all-purpose flour

1½ tsp. baking powder

¼ tsp. onion salt

3 Tbsp. margarine, softened

½ c. milk

1 Tbsp. snipped chives

Preheat oven to 450° F. Mix flour, baking powder, and onion salt in a bowl. Cut in softened margarine until like coarse crumbs. Make a well in the center of the mixture.

Add milk and chives all at once, then stir quickly just until the dough sticks together. Spoon out by rounded tablespoonfuls onto an ungreased cookie sheet.

Bake on an ungreased cookie sheet at 450° F. for 12 to 15 minutes. (Biscuits are done when top is golden).

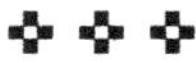

Cinnamon-Oat Bread 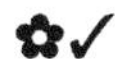

makes one loaf

The warmth of cinnamon and a hint of sweetness make this fiber-enhanced loaf perfect for hot buttered slices of toast.

- 1 c. milk, scalded
- 6 Tbsp. sugar
- 1 tsp. salt
- 3 Tbsp. margarine
- 1 packet active dry yeast
- 3 Tbsp. warm (110° F) water, test on wrist like baby formula
- ⅔ c. quick-cooking oats
- 4 tsp. cinnamon
- ⅛ tsp. nutmeg
- 1 egg
- 3 c. all-purpose flour (plus or minus half a cup)

Bring milk to boil in a saucepan, then stir in sugar, salt, and margarine. Set aside to cool. Meanwhile, add the yeast to the lukewarm water and set that aside to soften, about 10 minutes. In a blender or food processor, chop oats until texture is like cornmeal.

When yeast is softened and milk is lukewarm, stir one cup of the flour into the milk, beating well. Then add the chopped oats, yeast, cinnamon, nutmeg, and egg. Continue to stir in the flour until it is a moderately stiff dough. Turn out on a lightly floured surface, and knead until it is smooth and elastic, about 7 minutes.

Oil a bowl lightly with cooking oil. Place dough in bowl and oil top surface of dough. Cover and let rise in a warm place for 1½ hours (make sure it's not too hot or the yeast will die— the best temperature is about 80° F. to 85° F.)

Punch down dough with your fist, folding edges towards the center. Knead 4 or 5 times. Form dough into a ball. Cover and let the dough rest 10 minutes.

Shape in a loaf and place in a greased loaf pan, let rise til double, about 55-60 minutes. Bake in a pre-heated, 375° F. oven about 35 to 40 minutes (tap top with a fingernail— it should sound hollow when done. You can cover the bread with foil the last 15 minutes if it's browning too fast). Remove from the pan and cool on a wire rack.

Raisin-bread variation: Decrease the oats to ½ cup and add 1⅓ cup of raisins. (Soak in water for ten minutes to plump, then drain before adding).

Super-cinnamon swirl variation:

After the dough finishes its first rising, punch down and let rest five minutes. Meanwhile, combine ¼ c. sugar, 1 Tbsp. cinnamon, and a pinch of allspice. Roll out dough to a 9-inch by 12-inch rectangle. Brush with water, then sprinkle with the cinnamon-sugar mixture. Roll up, starting at the short end. Pinch to seal edges, and fold over ends. Place in loaf pan seam side down for the second rising. Let rise and bake same as Cinnamon-Oat bread recipe.

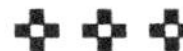

Georgia's Best Cornbread ✿✓

serves 5

¾ c. all-purpose flour
1¼ c. cornmeal
¼ c. sugar
4½ tsp. baking powder
¾ tsp. salt
2 eggs
1 c. milk
5 Tbsp. margarine or butter, melted

Grease a 9-inch square baking pan, or a 9-inch by 5-inch loaf pan. Preheat oven to 425° F. Combine the flour, corn meal, sugar, baking powder, and salt in a bowl. Make a well in the center. Add eggs, milk, and melted margarine all at once. Beat just until smooth (don't overbeat). Turn into the greased pan and bake at 425° F. for 30 minutes. Serve warm with butter and honey.

Tex-Mex Cornbread ✿

serves 5

This cornbread tastes like a tamale or tortilla, and is good with any Southwest-style main dish. Delicious with the traditional Mexican soup, Albondigas (see recipe in Soups and Stews).

Make just as you would the corn-bread recipe on this page, except: Use 2 cups of masa harina in place of the all-purpose flour and the cornmeal, and increase the milk to 1¼ cups. Add 3 Tbsp. of finely chopped red bell pepper for a colorful accent. Batter will be very thick, so you have to spread it out evenly in a greased 9-inch square baking pan. Bake at 425° F. for 30 minutes.

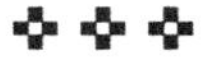

Traditional White Bread ✿✓

makes 3 loaves

Remember when the tantalizing aroma of Grandma's bread filled the kitchen while it baked to golden perfection? This version of the loaf has a delectable texture, but is lower in fat and sugar than many other recipes for white bread.

4 c. milk, scalded
¼ c. sugar
4 tsp. salt
3 Tbsp. stick butter or margarine
2 packets active dry yeast
½ c. warm (110° F) water
10 c. unbleached, all-purpose flour

10 c. unbleached, all-purpose flour (plus or minus half a cup)

Scald the milk in a saucepan, then stir in sugar, salt, and butter. Set aside to cool. Meanwhile, add the yeast to the lukewarm water and set that aside to soften, about 10 minutes.

When yeast is softened, stir three cups of the flour into the milk, beating well. Then add the yeast. Continue to stir in the flour until it is a moderately stiff dough (may take 9 to 11 cups of flour depending on the humidity of the air).

Turn the dough out on a lightly floured surface, and knead it vigorously until it is smooth, satiny, and elastic (and the gluten has developed), about 9 minutes.

Oil a bowl lightly with cooking oil. Place dough in bowl and oil top surface of dough. Cover with a damp cloth and let rise in a warm place for 1¼ hours (make sure it's not too hot or the yeast will die. The best temperature is about 82° F.)

Punch down dough with your fist, folding edges towards the center. Knead two or three times. Cut dough in three portions. Form each into a ball. Cover and let the dough rest ten minutes.

Shape into loaves and place in three greased 9 x 5 x 3 loaf pans. Cover and let rise until double, 55 to 65 minutes. Don't let it rise too long or the flour walls between the gas bubbles will get too thin and the bread may fall when it's baked. Brush top of loaf with an egg yolk mixed with a tablespoon of milk if you want a shiny crust.

Bake in a preheated, 375° F. oven about 45 minutes (tap the top of the bread with your fingernail, a hollow sound means it's done). You can cover the bread with foil the last 15 minutes if it's browning too fast.

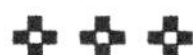

Wheat Flour and Nutrition

The wheat flour most commonly used today is not the flour Americans ate a century ago. As milling methods changed, so did the type of flour being produced. Some of these changes have not been for the better.

Flour milling and nutrient loss

There are several types of mills used by commercial enterprises to mill wheat into flour. The kind of mill that is used can affect the nutritional quality of the flour. Most commercial mills are hammer mills, blade mills or roller mills. Hammer mills smash the grains of wheat into particles with a hammer-like action. Blade mills chop it like a giant blender. High speed roller mills tear the grain between rotating cylinders. These milling techniques generate vast amounts of heat.

Heat is a major factor that adversely affects the amounts of certain nutrients in flour. In fact, at least seventeen different vitamins and minerals are typically lost in significant amounts during the milling of whole wheat into white flour.

Stone-ground mills, on the other hand, grind the grain between two surfaces. This action flakes layers off the wheat grain without heat. Unless a flour is specifically labeled "stone-ground," it is most likely milled by a cheaper method. Very little of the wheat flour we eat is stone-ground anymore.

According to data published in the *American Journal of Clinical Nutrition*, the amount of loss ranges from around 71% for vitamin B-6 and phosphorus, to about 87% for vitamin E and the trace element cobalt. A few of these nutrients are replaced in wheat flour that is "enriched," but most lost nutrients aren't replaced.

All-purpose Flour

Wheat germ is the innermost heart, or embryo, of a grain of wheat. The endosperm surrounds the germ. Wheat bran refers to the six layers that form the fibrous, indigestible outer coating of the grain. All-purpose white flour has the germ and bran removed. Only the endosperm is milled, and it is processed with approximately 30 chemicals to make it fluffier, more workable, or whiter.

If the flour is "bleached", it is chemically treated to make it slightly whiter in a process that destroys nutrients, including the anti-oxidant, vitamin E. That is why unbleached flour has a reputation for being more nutritious than bleached flour.

Enriched Flour

In the 1930's, after Americans began eating large amounts of white flour, surveys showed people were suffering dramatic deficiencies in some B vitamins and iron. Thanks to FDA intervention, "enriched" white flour came about. Four of the nutrients lost in milling and processing (thiamine, niacin, riboflavin, and iron) began to be replaced in the enriched version of white flour. Enriched white flour makes beautiful cakes and velvety smooth sauces, but is still not as nutrient-dense as stone-ground whole wheat flour.

Whole Wheat Flour

Whole wheat flour is made with all the parts of the wheat kernel, including the bran and the germ. Whole wheat flour, because of the oil in the germ, has a limited shelf life before becoming rancid. Heat and light can speed up the process of oxidation, which we call rancidity. It should always be stored in a cool, dark place or refrigerated.

Graham flour is just another name for whole wheat flour. It was named after Reverend Sylvester Graham who, in the late 1800's lectured churchgoers on the evils of white flour, featherbeds, and corsets.

Bulgar

Bulgar is wheat that is cracked into pieces rather than being milled, and therefore retains more nutrients. It is popular in the Middle East where it is used for pilaf or tabouleh. In the U.S., it is often called "cracked wheat."

Semolina

Semolina flour is ground from the heart of durum wheat. It's especially good for making pasta because the chemical structure allows it to keep its shape and not dissolve when boiled.

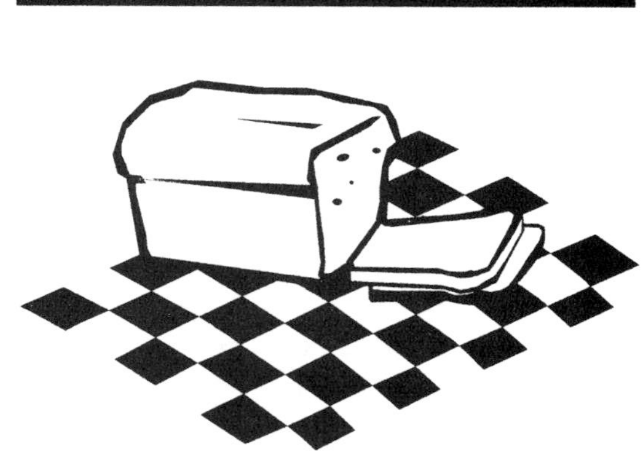

CAKES AND FROSTINGS

Quick Sherry Spice Cake ✿✓

makes 9 small servings

This moist cake is a delicious snack on crisp autumn evenings... it takes only 45 minutes to put together and bake, while it fills your kitchen with a wonderful spicy aroma!

1 c. all-purpose flour
½ c. sugar
½ tsp. cinnamon
½ tsp. allspice
½ tsp. baking soda
1 dash salt
1 egg
1 egg white
¼ c. water
2 Tbsp. sherry (not other white wine)
¼ c. molasses, unsulphured
½ Tbsp. butter, melted
whipped cream or vanilla ice cream (optional)

Grease one 9-inch square pan generously and preheat oven to 375° F. In medium mixing bowl, thoroughly combine the flour, sugar, cinnamon, allspice, baking soda and salt. Set aside.

In another bowl, whisk together the egg, egg white, water, sherry, and molasses. Melt butter in small pan or microwave, then whisk into the egg mixture. With a hand mixer at medium speed, beat together the egg mixture and dry ingredients, about 1 or 2 minutes.

Pour into greased pan and bake at 375° F. for 30 minutes, or until a toothpick in center comes out clean. Cool and slice into nine squares. Top each with whipped cream or vanilla ice cream and serve. *Calories per serving: 138*

Note: The alcohol in the sherry boils off during baking.

Dress it up: Place a doily or paper cutout on top of cake. Sift powdered sugar over paper. Carefully lift paper and your design of sugar will remain.

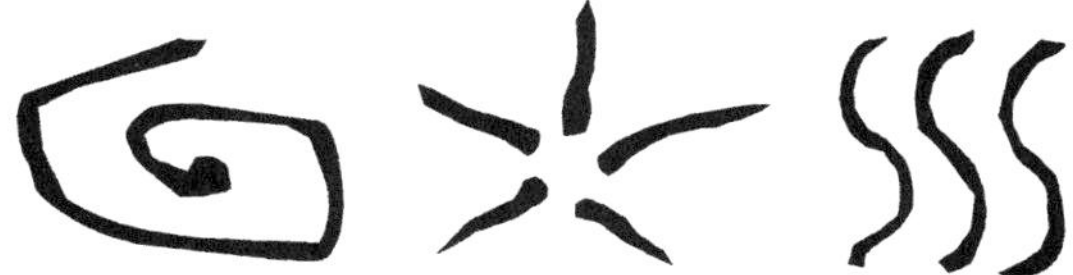

Easy Pastry Decorating

A ziplock plastic bag with the corner cut makes an excellent and disposable pastry bag. Cut off the lower corner of the bag and insert a metal pastry tip through the hole. Just be sure to use a large, heavy duty bag, not a little sandwich bag, especially not the ones with the pleated bottom. Plastic freezer bags work well. Fill the bag with the frosting, mashed potatoes, or whatever, and use. Squeeze the end just as you would a pastry tube. If you need to store it, press the contents away from the pastry tip, zip the top shut and stick it in the fridge. When you're done, remove the tip and toss the bag. A lot less mess than cleaning a cloth pastry bag!

Carrot-Coconut Cake ✿✓

serves 12

2 c. flour

1⅓ c. sugar

1½ tsp. baking soda

½ tsp. salt

2 tsp. cinnamon

3 eggs

⅓ c. vegetable oil

¾ c. lowfat milk

2 tsp. vanilla extract

2½ c. finely grated carrots

¾ c. finely chopped almonds

1¼ c. coconut, shredded, unsweetened ★

Grease and flour a 8-inch by 12-inch baking pan. Preheat oven to 375° F.

Thoroughly combine flour, sugar, soda, salt and cinnamon. In another bowl, beat eggs, oil, milk, and vanilla together until smooth. Add dry ingredients, mixing well. Stir in the carrots, almonds and coconut. Spoon into pan and bake at 375° F. for 45 minutes, or until center of cake springs back when lightly touched.

When cool, frost with Vanilla Cream Cheese Frosting and sprinkle with a little more shredded coconut, if desired. (Must be refrigerated if using a cream cheese frosting). *Calories per serving: 539*

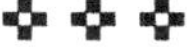

Maple Nut Chiffon Cake ✿✓

serves 8

6 Tbsp. real maple syrup (pure, 100%)

⅓ c. cold water

2 c. sifted all-purpose flour (measure after sifting)

¾ c. sugar

3 tsp. baking powder

1 tsp. salt

¾ c. light brown sugar, packed

½ c. salad oil

5 egg yolks

⅓ c. finely chopped nuts (see note)

1 c. egg whites (will be whites of 8 or 9 eggs)

½ tsp. cream of tartar

Stir to completely combine maple syrup and cold water.

Combine the measured flour with the sugar, baking powder, and salt. Stir in the brown sugar, mixing well. Make a well in the center. Pour the oil into the well, then the egg yolks, then the syrup water. With an electric mixer, beat until smooth. Stir in nuts.

For the next step, wash the beaters very well to remove all traces of oil and don't use a plastic bowl. (The tiniest amount of grease will keep the eggs from being fluffy enough). Beat the cupful of egg whites with the cream of tartar until very stiff peaks form. (To test: cut egg whites with a spatula or wide cake knife— it should make a clear path).

Gently fold in egg whites until batter is uniform. Pour into a clean, ungreased

10-inch tube pan. Bake at 350° F. for 1 hour. When done, remove from oven and immediately turn the pan upside down. Let cool for 1 hour, then cut cake loose from the side of the pan with a knife. Frost with Vanilla Cake Frosting or Brown Sugar Frosting. *Calories per serving: 847 to 870*

Note: Walnuts work best, if you can eat them, but almonds are delicious too. You can also simply leave out the nuts. If you have a little extra chopped nuts, sprinkle them on top of the frosting.

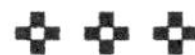

Granny's Graham Cracker Cake ✿

serves 8

⅔ c. margarine, at room temperature

1¾ c. sugar

2 eggs

2 tsp. vanilla

2⅓ c. all-purpose flour

2½ tsp. baking powder

1¼ tsp. salt

⅓ c. graham cracker crumbs ★

1¼ c. milk

Grease and flour two 8-inch cake pans. Preheat oven to 350° F.

Cream butter and sugar until light. Add eggs and vanilla, beating until fluffy. Combine dry ingredients in a large bowl, mixing well. Add milk to dry ingredients alternately with egg mixture while beating. Beat another minute, then pour into cake pans. While pans are on a flat surface, spin each pan so that batter spreads out from the center.

Place in oven and bake at 350° F. for 35 minutes or until top springs back when touched. Let cool before removing from pans. Frost with Brown Sugar Frosting. *Calories per serving: 850*

Note: You may find that making your own crumbs is better than buying packaged crumbs. Sometimes packaged crumbs have ingredients that the whole crackers don't have.

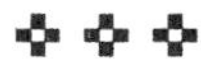

No-Acid Orange Cake ✿

serves 8

Making a tasty citrus cake without orange juice (which helps the batter rise) or artificial food coloring is a real challenge. This cake meets the challenge head on, and is surprisingly tender and flavorful.

2¼ c. all-purpose flour

3 tsp. baking powder

½ tsp. baking soda

¾ tsp. salt

⅔ c. unsalted butter, softened

1⅓ c. sugar

2 egg yolks

2 tsp. orange extract

¼ tsp. turmeric, optional (see note)

4 egg whites

1 c. minus 2 Tbsp. lowfat milk

Preheat oven to 350° F., then gather three mixing bowls. Grease and flour two 8-inch cake pans.

In the first mixing bowl, thoroughly combine flour, baking powder, baking soda, and salt.

In second mixing bowl, beat butter and sugar together. Add egg yolks and orange extract to sugar mixture while beating at medium speed with electric mixer. Add milk (and turmeric, if desired) alternately with dry ingredients while beating until uniform texture. Wash beaters very well to remove all traces of butter.

In the third bowl, beat egg whites at high speed until soft peaks form. Gently fold egg whites into batter. Spoon batter into cake pans and bake at 350° F. until toothpick in center comes out dry, about 30 to 35 minutes. Frost with Lemon Butter Frosting. *Calories per serving: 774*

Note: Turmeric is a mild spice that will add no noticeable flavor, but tint the food pale yellow. You can also use food coloring (1 drop red and 3 drops yellow) to tint the cake a pale orange.

Three-Vegetable Cake ✿✓

makes 9 small servings

Grandma Denson's small kitchen always smelled like fresh lemons, and as a child I watched with rapt attention as she would "just whip together a little something" whenever I visited. Nimbly mixing cake ingredients, she never measured, but always turned out the most heavenly treats. She would use whatever she had on hand, and much to my fascination, that often involved some pretty peculiar cake ingredients. This recipe is based on one of her "inventions" (a sly attempt, I suspect, to get me to eat more vegetables).

1 medium russet potato
3 Tbsp water or milk, approximately
½ c. finely shredded carrot
½ c. finely shredded zucchini
5 egg whites
1¼ tsp. vanilla
⅓ c. vegetable oil
1½ c. all purpose flour
1¼ c. sugar
1 tsp. baking powder
1 tsp. baking soda
2 tsp. cinnamon
½ tsp. salt

Peel potato, cut in 1-inch chunks and boil until completely soft and falling apart, about 20 minutes. Drain well. Mash potato or put through a potato ricer, then mix with water or milk until a smooth consistency, like soft mashed potatoes. Measure one-half cup into a bowl, add zucchini and carrot. Mix together and set aside. Preheat oven to 350° F. With an electric mixer, beat together egg whites, vanilla, and vegetable oil at medium speed, one minute. Add vegetables to the egg mixture and beat at low speed until blended. In a separate bowl, thoroughly combine the last six dry ingredients. Add the dry ingredients to the egg mixture a little at a time, while beating, until completely blended. Pour into a greased and floured 9-inch square cake pan.

Bake at 350° F. for 50 minutes or until toothpick in the center comes out clean. Cool about 10 minutes before removing from the pan. When cake is completely cooled, frost with Vanilla Cream Cheese Frosting, Orange Cream Cheese Frosting, or Vanilla Cake Frosting. *Calories per serving: 677 (cream cheese frosted) or 623* (if you use Vanilla Cake Frosting).

Cake should be refrigerated if using cream cheese frostings. You can also double the recipe: use a 13-inch by 9-inch pan (bake about 6 minutes longer), and frost as for a sheet cake. (See Sheet Cake Embellishments, pg. 96).

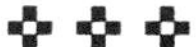

Pear Spice Cupcakes ✿✓

makes 24

3 ripe pears, peeled and sliced

¾ c. plus 2 Tbsp. water

6 Tbsp. brown sugar

3¾ c. all-purpose flour

1½ tsp. baking soda

1 tsp. salt

¾ tsp. baking powder

1½ tsp. cinnamon

¾ tsp. nutmeg

½ tsp. allspice

¾ c. margarine, softened

1½ c. sugar

3 eggs

In saucepan, combine pears, water, and brown sugar. Simmer covered for about 10 minutes, or until the pears are very soft. Remove from heat and puree pears in a blender or food processor. Set pear puree aside to cool.

Preheat oven to 350° F. Combine flour, baking soda, salt, baking powder, and spices, mixing well. Set aside.

With electric mixer, beat butter and sugar together, then beat in eggs at medium speed for two more minutes. Beat in the dry ingredients and pear puree alternately at low speed.

Pour into paper bake cups, filling each about three-quarters full. Bake at 350° F. for about 30 minutes, or until top of the cupcakes spring back when touched. Cool completely before frosting. Excellent with Vanilla Cake Frosting. *Calories per serving: 317*

Sheet Cake Embellishments

Here are some ideas to beautify that plain-jane frosted sheet cake:

Checkerboard Cake: Before frosting, cut cooled cake in equal squares. Divide vanilla frosting in half, tinting one half with food color, beet juice or turmeric. Frost each piece separately in a checkerboard pattern, then re-assemble. "Chess pieces" or "checkers" can be placed on the center of each piece of cake (use caramels or cut licorice, small foil-wrapped candies, mint gum drops, carob-coated mints, pieces of unwrapped salt water taffy, or tiny marshmallows.)

Wildflower Cake: In the center of a frosted cake make a small bouquet of edible flowers and parsley or mint, edged with a lace pattern of contrasting frosting. Johnny-jump-up violets have a pleasing floral taste. The Feb/Mar 1997 edition of *Herb Companion* (Interweave Press) lists many more edible flowers, including dianthus, broccoli flowers, pansy, and runner bean flowers. (Nasturtiums taste peppery. Chive flowers are edible but have an onion-y flavor). Be sure the flowers are pesticide-free.

Angel Cake ✿✓

serves 12

1 c. minus 2 Tbsp. all-purpose flour
¾ c. sugar
¼ tsp. salt
1½ c. egg whites (about 12 eggs)
1 tsp. cream of tartar
2 tsp. vanilla extract
¾ c. sugar

Preheat oven to 375° F. Sift (not stir) together the flour, ¾ c. sugar, and salt. Set aside for the moment.

With very clean beaters, beat egg whites, cream of tartar, and vanilla until soft peaks form. Beat in the remaining ¾ c. sugar until peaks are very stiff and glossy. Gradually fold in the flour mixture a little at a time.

Bake for 35 to 40 minutes at 375° F. (It's done if it springs back when touched). Turn upside down to cool. When cooled, remove from pan. *Calories per serving: 148 (unfrosted), 374 (frosted)*

Frost using Vanilla Cake Frosting with 1 c. unsweetened, shredded coconut ★ added, if desired. Or...

In a saucepan, bring 3 c. sugar and 1½ c. water to a boil. Cook until it reaches 226° F. Remove from heat and let cool to 110° F. Stir in 1 tsp. vanilla, a few drops of food coloring, and about 2½ c. powdered sugar. Pour over cake with a spoon, letting it run down sides. Let dry. Spoon on another coat. Top with "flowers" made of small marsh-mallows, snipped in half to form petals.

Tropical Gold Chiffon Cake ✿✓

serves 12

2 c. all-purpose flour
1½ c. sugar
3 tsp. baking powder
1 tsp. salt
½ c. vegetable oil
4 egg yolks (use large eggs)
¾ c. milk
1½ tsp. vanilla
⅛ tsp. turmeric
½ tsp. cream of tartar
9 egg whites (use large eggs)
toasted nuts or coconut ★

Preheat oven to 325° F. and gather two bowls and a 10-inch tube pan. In the first bowl, sift (not stir) together flour, sugar, baking powder, and salt. With electric mixer, beat in the oil, then egg yolks. Beat in the milk, vanilla and turmeric until satiny smooth.

Clean beaters very well to remove all traces of oil. In the second bowl, beat together the cream of tartar and egg whites until very stiff peaks form. Pour the yellow batter over the egg whites and gently fold in. Carefully scoop batter into the tube pan (don't use any grease on the pan).

Bake for 1 hour and 10 minutes at 325° F. (It's done if it springs back when touched). Turn upside down to cool. Frost when cool with Vanilla Cake Frosting, sprinkle toasted chopped cashews or coconut on top of cake. *Calories per serving: 520* .

Carob Cupcakes ✿✓

makes 20-24

½ c. margarine
1½ c. sugar
1 tsp. vanilla
1 egg
2 egg whites
¾ c. carob powder
1¾ c. all-purpose flour
1 tsp. baking soda
1 tsp. baking powder
⅛ tsp. salt
⅛ tsp. cream of tartar
1¾ c. milk

Cream margarine sugar and vanilla until fluffy. Blend in the eggs and egg whites. In another bowl, mix together carob powder, flour, baking soda, baking powder, salt, and cream of tartar. Preheat oven to 350° F.

To dry ingredients, alternately add milk and egg mixture while beating smooth at medium speed. Beat well about 1 minute more. Divide batter among 20 to 24 paper bake cups, filling at least two-thirds full, and bake at 350° F. for 30 minutes or until center springs back when touched. Frost when cool with Cooked Coconut Frosting *(calories per serving: 266)* or Vanilla Cake Frosting *(calories per serving: 300).*

Note: These freeze quite well.

Almond Cupcakes  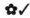

makes 24

¾ c. margarine (stick kind)
1½ c. sugar
1¼ tsp. almond extract
1 tsp. vanilla extract
1 egg
4 egg whites
2 c. all-purpose flour
1 Tbsp. baking powder
1 tsp. salt
1 c. milk
¼ c. chopped almonds
½ c. chopped dates

Preheat oven to 375° F. Cream margarine, sugar, almond extract, and vanilla until fluffy. Blend in the egg and egg whites until uniform consistency.

In another bowl, mix together flour, baking powder, and salt. To the egg mixture, add dry ingredients and milk alternately while beating at medium speed with electric mixer. Continue to beat one minute more. Stir in chopped almonds and dates.

Fill paper bake cups about ¾-full with batter. Bake at 375° F. for 20 to 22 minutes. Tops will be golden brown. Cool completely before frosting with Vanilla Cake Frosting. *Calories per frosted cupcake: 300*

Holiday variation: Give these a festive look by adding a couple of tablespoons of chopped maraschino cherries (if you can eat them) to the cake batter. Bits of dried apricot or raisins work well too. Watch out for sorbates and sulfites on dried and glacé fruit. For sources of preservative-free dried fruit, see Appendix B.

Jam-filled variation: Heat ¼ cup of preservative-free apricot, blackberry or blueberry jam in a saucepan until it is liquid. Add ¼ tsp. baking soda and stir. (Jam will be frothy. The soda helps neutralize fruit acids). Remove from heat and stir 2 or 3 minutes until foam subsides. Let jam cool while making cupcake batter. To assemble: Fill paper bake cups with a heaping tablespoon of batter, then drop a teaspoon of jam into center. Continue to fill bake cup ¾ full, then bake and frost as for main recipe.

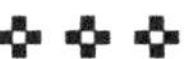

Vanilla Cake Frosting 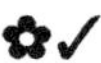

frosts two 9-inch layers, or 24 cupcakes

½ c. softened butter or margarine
4 c. powdered sugar, divided
2 tsp. vanilla extract
¼ c. low-fat milk

Cream the softened butter or margarine with two cups of the powdered sugar. When light and fluffy, add the vanilla extract and milk. Beat in the remaining two cups of powdered sugar a little at a time, to make the mixture spreadable and just a bit thinner than you want it to be. (The frosting will thicken a bit as you work).

Orange Cream Cheese Frosting ✿

frosts two 8-inch layers

16 oz. cream cheese, softened
½ c. unsalted butter, softened
1 c. powdered sugar
1½ tsp. vanilla
¼ tsp. orange extract
2 tsp. grated orange peel
food coloring (optional)

With electric mixer, blend cream cheese and butter until smooth and creamy. Gradually add the remaining ingredients while beating at medium speed. Add coloring last, if desired. (Some people are sensitive to yellow #5, so check labels).

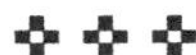

Lemon Butter Frosting ✿

frosts two 9-inch layers

½ c. softened butter
3½ c. powdered sugar
¼ tsp. vanilla extract
¾ tsp. lemon extract
1¼ tsp. freshly grated lemon peel
⅛ tsp. turmeric
¼ c. milk

Cream the softened butter together with 2 cups of the sugar. When fluffy, add vanilla extract, turmeric, and milk. Add remaining powdered sugar while beating, to make the mixture spreadable. (If you wish to omit the lemon peel, increase the lemon extract to 1½ tsp).

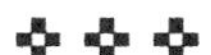

Vanilla Cream Cheese Frosting ✿✓

frosts two 8-inch layers

16 oz. cream cheese, softened
½ c. unsalted butter, softened
1½ c. powdered sugar
1¾ tsp. vanilla

Let cream cheese and butter come to room temperature. In a bowl, mix the cream cheese and butter with an electric mixer until smooth. Gradually add the sugar and vanilla while beating.

When smooth and uniform consistency, spread on cake. (It spreads best at room temperature, but you can make it ahead, refrigerate, and use it later). The finished cake should be refrigerated.

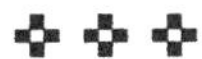

Cooked Coconut Frosting ✿✓

frosts tops of two 8-inch layers or 24 cupcakes

1 egg
1 6-oz. can of evaporated milk (not condensed)
⅔ c. sugar
¼ c. margarine or butter
1½ c. shredded coconut, unsweetened ★
⅓ c. chopped cashews or almonds

Beat egg slightly and add to a saucepan with the milk, sugar, and margarine. Cook and stir about 10 minutes over medium heat until thickened and bubbly. Stir in coconut and nuts. Remove from heat and set aside to cool. When cooled, about 20 minutes, spread on cake or cupcakes.

Note: Pecans work well too, if you can tolerate them. Avoid coconut treated with sorbates or metabisulfite.

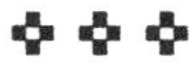

No-Fat Spice Frosting ✿✓

frosts 24 cupcakes

For those who are watching their weight (or total fat intake) but just have to have a little treat, try this frosting on Pear Spice Cupcakes. Made with this frosting, the cupcakes are only about 250 calories each—40% less than most cupcakes.

2 egg whites
1¼ c. sugar
¼ c. maple syrup
¼ c. cold water
dash salt
¼ tsp. cinnamon

Place all ingredients in top of double boiler (but not over boiling water yet). With an electric mixer, beat together until well blended. Then place over the boiling water, but don't let the bottom of the pot touch the water. Continue to beat the ingredients constantly, for seven full minutes. Stiff peaks will form. Remove from over the water and beat until spreading consistency.

Note: This frosting, when set, tends to be slightly stiff (more like an ornamental frosting), rather than very soft like butter-based frostings. (It works fine for decorating). Thinned a bit after cooking, it can be poured over an angel or bundt cake as a glaze.

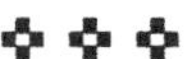

Brown Sugar Frosting ✿✓

frosts two 9-inch layers

A delicious, rich, old-fashioned frosting.

½ c. butter (not margarine)
1 c. light brown sugar
¼ c. milk
3¼ c. powdered sugar

Melt butter in a saucepan over medium heat, being careful not to scorch. Add the brown sugar and bring to a rolling boil (mixture will be thick and fluffy). Continue cooking about 30 seconds more. Remove from the heat and set aside to cool 10 minutes. When cooled, add milk, mixing until smooth. Beat in powdered sugar until spreading consistency (may be a little more or less than given amount).

Frost cake when completely cooled. (For a decorative touch, use a long knife or spatula to smooth frosting over cake, then sprinkle finely chopped nuts on top. Use a pastry tube to pipe a decorative top edging).

COOKIES

Jamaican Cashew Cookies ✿✓

makes 48

⅔ c. margarine
1 c. light brown sugar
½ c. sugar
1 tsp. vanilla extract
½ tsp. cinnamon
½ tsp. allspice
½ tsp. dried ginger
½ tsp. anise seed, crushed
2 eggs

2 c. flour
1 tsp. baking soda
1 c. quick-cooking oats
1 c. salted cashews, chopped

Preheat oven to 350° F.

Melt margarine. In a bowl, add melted margarine to sugars, mixing well until no dry sugar remains. Add vanilla, spices and eggs, mixing thoroughly until uniform consistency.

In separate bowl, mix flour and baking soda thoroughly. Add oats and cashews. Stir liquid ingredients into dry ingredients and mix well. Drop batter on greased baking sheets by tablespoons, leaving two inches between. Bake until golden, about 10 to 12 minutes. *Calories per cookie: 93*

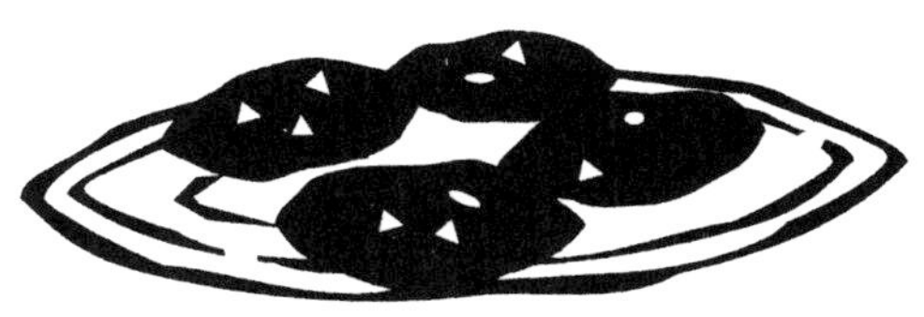

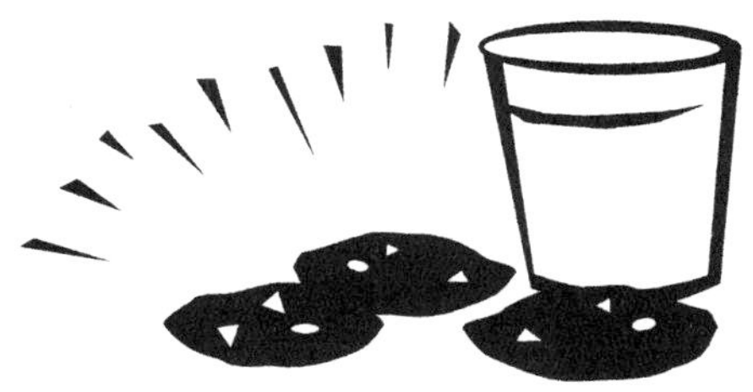

Dutch Carob Cookies ✿✓

makes 40

1 c. all-purpose flour
4½ Tbsp. carob powder
½ tsp. baking soda
¼ tsp. salt
¼ tsp. mace

½ c. sugar
¼ c. light brown sugar, packed
⅓ c. butter
¼ c. margarine
2 egg whites
3 Tbsp. low-fat milk
1¼ tsp. vanilla extract
¼ c. chopped nuts, optional

Preheat oven to 375° F.

Combine flour, carob powder, baking soda, salt, and mace in a mixing bowl. In another bowl, beat sugars, butter, and margarine until fluffy. Add egg whites, milk, and vanilla, beating well. Add egg and sugar mixture to dry ingredients, mixing well. Stir in nuts if desired. Drop batter by rounded teaspoonfuls onto a greased or non-stick cookie sheet. Bake at 375° F. for 8 to 10 minutes. *Calories per cookie: 60*

Versatile Butterscotch Cookies ✿✓

makes 24

½ c. butter
⅔ c. light brown sugar
1 egg
1⅓ c. all-purpose flour
1 tsp. baking soda
1 tsp. vanilla
¼ c. butterscotch chips, optional ★

Melt butter in a medium saucepan. Remove from heat and add brown sugar, mixing until sugar is smooth and lump-free. Add egg and vanilla, beating until smooth.

Mix together flour and baking soda, then stir into batter. Chill batter in the refrigerator about ten minutes. Stir in butterscotch chips if desired.

Bake at 375° F. for 7-8 minutes on an ungreased cookie sheet. Remove at once. *Calories per cookie: 84*

Note: These cookies are good just plain, but you can let the kids decorate them with sugar sprinkles, or add the following instead of the butterscotch chips: Golden raisins, chopped dates, dried black currants, chopped almonds or cashews, carob chips or white chocolate chips (for those who can tolerate white chocolate).

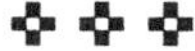

Holiday Gingerbread Cookies ✿✓

makes 36

½ c. margarine
½ c. sugar
¼ tsp. salt
½ c. molasses
2 Tbsp. milk
1 egg
1 tsp. baking soda
3 tsp. dried ginger
½ tsp. cinnamon
¼ tsp. allspice
2½ c. flour

Melt margarine and pour into a mixing bowl. Add sugar, salt and molasses, combining well. Stir in milk and egg until even consistency. Add baking soda, ginger, cinnamon, allspice, mixing well after each addition. Stir in the flour, mixing until even consistency.

Refrigerate dough for 3 hours. Roll out chilled dough about ¼-inch thick on a floured surface and cut shapes. Place about half an inch apart on a greased or non-stick cookie sheet. Bake at 375° F. for 6 to 7 minutes. *Calories per cookie: 80*

Wreath variation: Roll the dough a bit thinner, then use small, leaf-shaped hors d'oeuvre cutters to cut out mini-cookies. Overlap leaves in a circle to make wreaths, pressing and sealing together with milk. (After baking and air drying, wreaths can be decorated and hung on ribbons).

Orange and Date Pinwheels ✿

makes 45

½ c. chopped dates
1 tsp. orange peel, finely grated (or ¼ tsp. orange extract)
½ c. water
¼ c. light brown sugar, packed

2 c. all-purpose flour
½ tsp. baking soda
⅛ tsp. cream of tartar
¼ tsp. salt
⅓ c. margarine or butter
½ c. light brown sugar, packed
¼ c. sugar
2 egg whites
½ tsp. orange extract
¼ tsp. vanilla
3 tsp. milk or water

In saucepan combine dates, orange peel, water, and ¼ cup brown sugar. Bring to boil and simmer about 7 minutes, or until mixture thickens. Remove and set aside to cool.

Thoroughly combine flour, baking soda, cream of tartar, and salt. Cream together the margarine and sugars, then beat in the egg whites, orange extract, vanilla and milk. Mix together the dry ingredients and the egg mixture to make a stiff dough.

Roll out dough on a floured surface to a thickness of about ¼-inch. Try to achieve general shape of a rectangle (this may require some cutting and re-rolling of pieces). Spread filling on dough and roll up. Wrap in wax paper and chill thoroughly, at least 3 hours.

Cut slices off roll with a sharp knife, about ¼-inch thick. Place on a greased baking sheet (or a non-stick one), and bake at 400° F. for 8 to 10 minutes. Cool on wire rack. *Calories per cookie:* 57

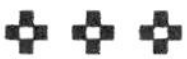

Grandma's Sugar Cookies ✿✓

makes 3 dozen

¾ c. margarine
¾ c. sugar
1 egg
1 Tbsp. vanilla
1 Tbsp. milk
2 c. flour
2 tsp. baking powder
¼ tsp. salt

Beat sugar and softened margarine until fluffy. Add egg, vanilla and milk, beating until thoroughly mixed. Mix dry ingredients together, then add to batter.

After mixing, chill 3 hours before rolling out ¼-inch thick. Cut in desired shapes with cookie cutters, sprinkle with colored sugar for holiday treats. Bake at 350° F. for 7-9 minutes until slightly brown around edges. Cool on racks. *Calories per cookie: 78*

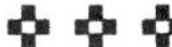

Holiday Cutout Stars ✿

makes 18 to 36 cookies

I've seen many versions of this cookie, but my favorite is this old recipe. Before the invention of margarine cooks used liberal amounts of real butter, which made their cookies rich and mellow. I've updated this one to reduce some of the fat and calories, but retain all the buttery flavor.

2¼ c. all-purpose flour
½ tsp. salt
½ c. margarine
½ c. real butter
1 c. sugar
1 egg
1 tsp. vanilla extract
⅓ c. pear ★ or other jam (see note)
1 large & 1 small star-shape cutter

Mix flour and salt, then set aside. Melt butter and margarine together. Add sugar to butter mixture and blend well. Beat in egg and vanilla with electric mixer. Gradually beat in flour mixture.

Divide dough in half and chill both halves 30 minutes or until firm enough to roll. (Preheat oven to 350° F. and have cookie sheets ready).

On a lightly floured surface, roll out half of the dough at a time to about an ⅛ of an inch thick. Cut out large stars, leaving 1 inch between cookies on sheet. Bake for 8 to 10 minutes, just til slightly golden on edges. Roll out other half of dough, cutting large stars, then cut small stars from the center of each large star (works best to do this while large stars are on cookie sheet). Bake for 8 to 10 minutes. Watch to avoid scorching.

Heat jam in small saucepan until melted (seedless jam is best). Brush center tops of whole cookies with hot jam. Place cutout cookies on top of whole cookies, staggering the star points. Cool and store with wax paper between layers. *Calories per cookie: varies from around 100 to 200, depending on size.*

Almond/apricot variation: Add ¼ tsp. almond extract and ¼ c. chopped almonds to the dough. Use apricot jam, and dust tops of cookies with powdered sugar, forced through a tea strainer with a spoon.

Note: This recipe is fun to vary. Any jam or jelly may be used. Pear, blueberry, or blackberry jam works well. (If you need to reduce the jam's acidity, add ⅛ tsp. of baking soda when you heat it. Stir for minute or so. The foam subsides as it cools, and won't affect the taste or appearance). Try colored frosting, melted caramel candies, or melted carob or butterscotch chips between the cookies.

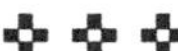

Nutty Blondies ✿✓

makes 16

If you long for the chewy goodness of brownies, these will make you forget your romance with chocolate!

½ c. unsalted butter
1¾ c. light brown sugar

1 egg
2 egg whites
1 Tbsp. vanilla extract
1½ c. all-purpose flour
3 tsp. baking powder
¾ tsp. salt
½ c. chopped cashews (or pecans if they don't bother you)

Preheat oven to 350° F. and cut wax paper or oiled parchment to fit inside of an 8-inch square pan. Coat pan with butter or margarine and line pan bottom and sides with wax paper. (Omit wax paper for non-stick pan).

Measure brown sugar into large mixing bowl and add melted butter. Mix well with large spoon until no dry brown sugar remains. Stir in vanilla, egg and egg whites, mixing well until batter is an even consistency. Sift flour, salt, and baking powder together, then stir into to the sugar mixture. Stir in nuts. Pour into baking pan. Bake at 350° F. for 40 to 45 minutes, until a toothpick in center comes out clean. When cool, turn upside down to remove from pan and cut into squares. *Calories per cookie: 184*

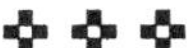

Low-Fat Graham-Almond Bars

makes 16

3 egg whites
1 tsp. vanilla extract
1 tsp. unsulphured molasses
½ c. sugar
5 Tbsp. light brown sugar, packed
¼ tsp. baking soda
3 Tbsp. all-purpose flour
14 square graham crackers, crushed (see note) ★
¼ c. finely chopped almonds

Preheat oven to 350° F., and grease and flour a 9-inch square pan. With electric beater, beat eggs whites until frothy, about 30 seconds. Beat in vanilla and molasses. In separate bowl, combine sugar, brown sugar, baking soda and flour. When uniformly mixed, stir in crumbs and almonds. Gently fold dry ingredients into the egg mixture. Batter will be very thick. Spoon the batter into the greased pan. Bake 25 minutes. Let cool about 20 minutes then cut into bars while still slightly warm. *Calories per cookie: 89*

Note: To crush graham crackers to fine crumbs, place a few crackers between sheets of wax paper and roll with a rolling pin.

Baking Powder Tip

If your baked goods don't rise as they should, check the expiration date on your baking powder. It may be too old to work properly. Another trick— put a teaspoon in a cup of very hot water. It should fizz if it's still okay to use.

Glazed Date Bars ✿✓

makes about 18

1 c. light brown sugar
½ c. margarine (at room temperature)
1½ c. all-purpose flour
½ tsp. baking soda
½ tsp. salt
¼ tsp. ground cinnamon
1⅓ c. quick-cooking oats
1 Tbsp. water

Filling:
¼ c. sugar
1 Tbsp. cornstarch
1 c. water
2 c. chopped dates ★

Glaze:
¾ c. powdered sugar
milk

Grease a 9-inch by 12-inch baking pan with margarine. Cream together the brown sugar and margarine. Add the flour, soda, salt and cinnamon stirring them into the brown sugar mixture. Add oats and water, mixing until it has a uniform crumb texture. Set aside.

For filling, combine sugar and cornstarch in a saucepan, mixing well. Stir in the water and dates. Cook while stirring, over medium heat, until the mixture is thickened. Remove from heat to slightly cool. Pat half the crumb mixture in the greased pan. Top with cooked filling. Mix the remaining half of the crumbs with about 2 teaspoons more water, and pat those over the top of the filling. Bake at 350° F. for 35 minutes. Let cool slightly before cutting.

When cooled, mix powdered sugar with a little milk to make a thick paste. Use a pastry tube with a small tip to make diagonal stripes of glaze across each bar. Or, use a little more milk and drip a design from a spoon. *Calories per cookie: 244*

Note: You can substitute the same amount of dried currants, raisins, or any dried fruit you can tolerate, for the dates.

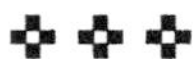

Frosted Carob Brownies 

makes 12

Brownies:
10 Tbsp. butter or margarine (½ c. plus 2 Tbsp.)
1 c. sugar
2 Tbsp. milk
2 eggs
⅔ c. all-purpose flour
6 Tbsp. carob powder
1½ tsp. baking powder
dash salt
½ c. chopped, dry roasted almonds

Frosting:
¼ c. butter (not margarine)
½ c. brown sugar
2 Tbsp. milk
1½ c. powdered sugar

Preheat oven to 350° F. Melt the 10 Tbsp. of butter and beat in the sugar until well blended. Beat in milk. Beat in eggs and egg white. Set aside.

Sift together flour, carob, baking powder, and salt. Add egg mixture to the dry ingredients, beating well. Stir in nuts. Pour into a greased and floured 9-inch square baking pan. Bake at 350° F. for 30 minutes, or until toothpick in center comes out clean. Let cool.

To make frosting: Melt butter in a saucepan over medium heat, being careful not to scorch. Add the brown sugar and bring to a rolling boil (mixture will be thick and fluffy). Continue cooking about 30 seconds more. Remove from heat and set aside to cool about 10 minutes. When cooled, add milk, mixing until smooth.

Beat in powdered sugar until spreading consistency (may be a little more or less than given amount). Frost brownies when completely cooled, then cut into 12 bars. *Calories per cookie: 349*

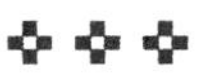

Crispy Peanut Butter Treats ✿✓

makes about 18 bars

My neighbor Corrine Blanding gave me her recipe for these chewy bars years ago. They are so good, I just couldn't resist including the recipe, even though not everyone with IC can eat peanuts. They are bound to become your kids' favorites!

1 c. sugar

1 c. light corn syrup

1 c. peanut butter ★

6½ c. Rice Krispies (see note)

¼ c. chopped peanuts, chopped cashews, or dried black currants, optional

In a large saucepan mix sugar and corn syrup. Heat and stir over a low flame until sugar is completely dissolved. Continue cooking and stirring. As soon as it comes to a rolling boil, remove from the heat. (Boiling too long will make it rock hard).

Quickly stir in peanut butter and chopped ingredients. As soon as it is well mixed, quickly stir in rice krispies. Promptly turn out into a 9-inch by 13-inch baking dish. Press down with back of a spoon or spatula. Let cool slightly, then cut in bars. *Calories per cookie: 173*

Note: If you are at all allergic, be careful of cereals with BHA and BHT. See Appendix B for sources of preservative-free cereals.

Kids' variations: Kids love these bars made with M&M's, or carob chips and butterscotch chips, instead of chopped nuts. They also like these topped with chocolate: melt chocolate chips in a double boiler and spread on top of bars, let cool before cutting.

Carob-frosted variation: You can also top these with a delicious carob frosting. Mix 3 Tbsp. carob powder, 1 Tbsp. melted butter, and 3 Tbsp. sugar. Heat and spread over cookies. Let cool, then cut.

Coconut and White Chocolate Bars ✿

makes 16

For the lucky people with IC who can tolerate white chocolate, these rich tropical treats are irresistible.

¼ c. butter or margarine, melted
¾ c. graham cracker crumbs ★
1 c. white (chocolate) baking chips ★
1 c. coconut, shredded, unsweetened ★
⅓ c. chopped salted cashews
1 14-oz. can sweetened, condensed (not evaporated) milk

Preheat oven to 350° F. Coat a 9-inch square baking pan with melted butter. Sprinkle graham cracker crumbs evenly in bottom of pan. Top with white chips, then coconut, then chopped nuts. Pour the milk over everything, then bake for 30 minutes. Cut into bars when cooled. *Calories per cookie: 256*

Note: Several companies make white chocolate morsels, but check the package carefully for artificial additives.

Also, it is better to make crumbs of graham crackers than to buy the crumbs already made. The ready-made crumbs often have more preservatives, and sometimes added spices or flavors. (To make crumbs of graham crackers, roll a few at a time between sheets of wax paper, pressing down with the rolling pin; or chop in a food processor).

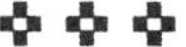

Peanut Butter Oatmeal Cookies ✿✓

makes about 48

½ c. unsalted butter
½ c. smooth peanut butter ★
¾ c. sugar
1 c. light brown sugar, packed
½ tsp. cinnamon
1 tsp. salt
1 egg
1 egg white
4 Tbsp. milk
1 tsp. vanilla
1¾ c. flour, all-purpose
1 tsp. baking soda
1⅓ c. rolled oats

Preheat oven to 350° F. Stir melted butter and peanut butter together until uniform consistency. Set aside.

Combine sugars, salt and cinnamon in a large mixing bowl. Add peanut butter mixture and stir until mixture is a soft, even consistency.

Stir in egg and egg white, then vanilla and milk. Mix thoroughly with spoon or electric mixer. In a separate bowl, combine flour, baking soda, and rolled oats. Stir dry ingredients into the batter, mixing thoroughly.

Drop dough by rounded table-spoonfuls onto a baking sheet, spacing them about two inches apart. Bake until golden brown, about 15 minutes. Store in an airtight container when cooled. *Calories per cookie: 86*

LUNCHES AND SNACKS

Hot Tuna Muffins ✓

serves 2

2 Tbsp. soft margarine

1 tsp. dried chervil

½ tsp. onion salt

⅛ tsp. pepper

1 6-oz. can flaked tuna, packed in water

¼ c. celery, finely chopped (see note)

2 English muffins, split

2 slices Muenster cheese

Mix softened margarine, chervil, onion salt, and pepper. Stir in drained tuna and celery, blending with a fork. Split each muffin and spread with the tuna mixture. Top with a slice of Muenster cheese. Toast until cheese is hot and bubbly. (Mozzarella also works well, and 2 tsp. fresh parsley can be used instead of dried chervil).

Note: For low-oxalate, chop fresh broccoli stalks fine to make a crunchy substitute for celery.

Grilled Turkey Sandwiches

serves 2

4 slices whole wheat bread

slices of Velveeta

slices of cooked turkey

1 bell pepper, cut in rings

2 Tbsp. snipped chives (see note)

margarine or butter

Spread four bread slices with margarine. Top 2 bread slices with velveeta, chives, bell pepper, then turkey. Top with remaining bread slices and spread margarine on the outsides of both bread sandwiches. Cook in skillet on medium heat until browned, turning to brown each side.

Note: If you wish to omit the chives, sprinkle onion salt on the margarine-spread bread slices.

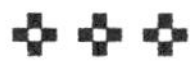

Fisherman's Pita Sandwich ✓

serves 2

1 6-oz. can tuna in water

1 Tbsp. olive oil

⅛ tsp black pepper (optional)

¼ tsp. garlic powder

¼ tsp. salt

¼ c. shredded lettuce

⅓ c. cottage cheese

½ tsp. dried dill

1 Tbsp. sunflower seeds (see note)

2 pita bread pockets

Drain tuna, squeezing moisture out. In bowl, combine olive oil, pepper (if desired), garlic powder and salt. Add flaked tuna and mix well with a fork. Fill pita bread with tuna, top with lettuce. In a bowl, mix cottage cheese, dill and sunflower seeds. Top tuna and lettuce with cottage cheese mixture.

Note: Be sure seeds don't have sulfites or hydrolyzed vegetable protein.

Snack Mix ✿

makes about 2¼ cups

1 c. salted cashews

1 c. pretzel sticks ★

½ c. dried currants or raisins

¼ c. sunflower seeds

Mix all ingredients together in a bowl and serve.

IC-Style Quesadillas 

serves 4

These are good to eat with hearty soups, especially Mexican Black Bean Soup. Or they just make great snacks!

4 corn tortillas

8 slices Muenster cheese

3 Tbsp. chopped chives or dash onion salt

Sprinkle a few drops of water on tortillas if they have been in the refrigerator awhile, otherwise keep dry. Stack tortillas on ceramic microwave-safe plate and microwave on high for about 20 seconds, just enough to get tortillas warm and able to roll without cracking.

Separate, place cheese in center of each tortilla, sprinkle with onion salt or chopped chives if desired. Roll up and microwave 20 seconds to melt cheese.

Seasoned Roasted Almonds 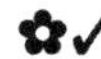

makes 1 cup

1 c. blanched almonds

2 Tbsp margarine

1½ tsp. onion salt

¼ tsp. garlic powder

¼ tsp. marjoram, crushed

Melt margarine over medium heat. Add almonds and cook while stirring about 3 or 4 minutes until they are a golden brown. Remove to paper towels, drain briefly and cool about five or ten minutes. Put in a ziplock bag with the remaining ingredients. Shake to coat. Serve as appetizers or snacks, warm or cold. (These will keep for quite awhile, even if not refrigerated).

Why Won't the Popcorn Pop?

It can be hard to get popcorn to pop if it's old and has lost its moisture. It needs to have just a tiny bit of water in the kernel. If you have old, dried out popcorn, try putting it in lukewarm water for six or seven minutes. Then take it out, dry it on a clean towel and try popping it.

Garlic Popcorn ✿

makes about 8 cups

Most "microwave bag" popcorn has additives that give me a bladder-symptom flare, so I buy the old-fashioned kernels and use a cheap microwavable popper and plain corn oil. We love this tasty variation.

½ c. unpopped popcorn

3 Tbsp. butter or margarine

¼ tsp. to ½ tsp. garlic powder

salt

Mix garlic powder into the butter then melt the butter in a small pan or in a microwave. Make popcorn as you usually do then pour the melted butter over popcorn. Toss, then salt as usual.

Lower-Fat variation: Air-pop the popcorn, then spray it lightly with olive oil cooking spray while tossing. Mix ½ tsp. salt and ¼ tsp. garlic powder in a small bowl and sprinkle over popcorn.

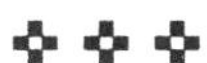

Vermont-Style Maple Popcorn ✿

serves 4

Kids love this yummy traditional New England snack. It can be stored for quite awhile, but you'll be tempted to eat it all right away!

1 c. popcorn kernels, unpopped

10 Tbsp. margarine

1⅓ c. maple syrup

¼ c. sugar

¼ tsp. salt

⅛ tsp. baking soda

½ tsp. baking powder

Make popcorn as you usually would, and spread the kernels out in a single layer on a 12-inch by 18-inch rimmed cookie sheet that has been coated with non-stick cooking spray. Melt the margarine in a saucepan, then add maple syrup, sugar, and salt. Using a candy thermometer, heat the mixture to 240° F while stirring. Remove from heat and immediately stir in the baking soda and baking powder. Drizzle the foamy mixture over popcorn. Bake for 1 hour at 200° F. Remove from oven and let cool for 20 minutes before removing popcorn from the cookie sheet. Scrape off with a rubber spatula, or break pieces off. Let dry on a cool surface for several hours or overnight. Then store in an airtight container or serve.

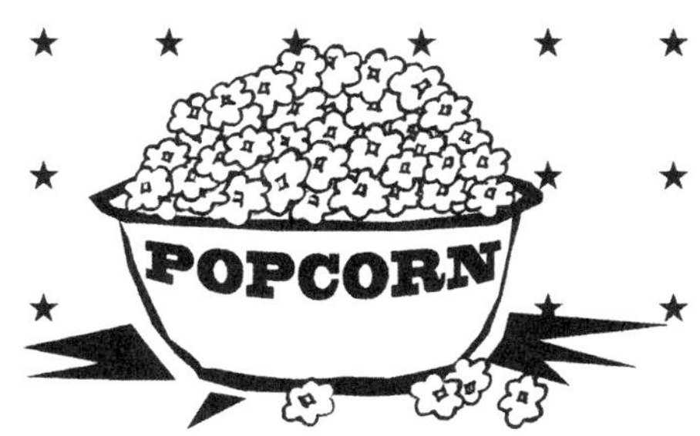

Fruit Leather ✿

To make pear, blueberry, or blackberry fruit leather, first pick only very ripe fruit. (Not only does ripe fruit work best, but it is generally lower in acid). Puree the fruit and strain out seeds if using blackberries. Spread on a rimmed cookie sheet that has been lined with wax paper or sprayed with non-stick cooking spray. Tilt the pan so the puree spreads out to no more than ¼-inch thick. Place in the oven at no more than 140° F. and heat with the door propped slightly open for moisture to escape. Fruit leather is done when it is dry but slightly sticky and can be peeled easily. For fruit that is too thin and runny, you can add a little mashed banana if bananas don't bother you. You can also sweeten it with a little honey. (If you use honey, a couple of teaspoons for each cup of puree will do the trick).

The fruit leather you make at home won't look like commercially prepared ones, which have additives such as ascorbic acid (vitamin C) or citric acid to keep the fruit puree from turning brown. There's nothing unhealthful about brown fruit leather, it just doesn't look as attractive. It looks, well... like leather.

Candied Almonds 

makes 1¼ cups

¾ c. sugar
¼ c. water
1 tsp. cinnamon
⅛ tsp. nutmeg
⅛ tsp. salt
1¼ c. whole almonds

Add all ingredients except nuts to a saucepan and heat to 240° F. on a candy thermometer. Quickly add almonds and stir just until coated. Immediately turn out on wax paper or aluminum foil, push nuts apart quickly. When cool, store in an airtight container.

Salt Water Taffy 

makes about ¾ pound

1 c. sugar
½ c. light corn syrup
¾ tsp. salt
¾ c. water
1 Tbsp. margarine
¼ tsp. lemon, orange or peppermint extract *or*, ½ tsp. vanilla
4 or 5 drops food coloring (see note)

Coat kitchen scissors and a 9-inch square baking pan with margarine. In a saucepan, combine the sugar, corn syrup, salt and water. Cook over medium heat, stirring, until sugar dissolves. Using a candy thermometer, cook to 260° F. without stirring. Remove from heat and mix in remaining ingredients.

Pour in buttered pan, let cool until comfortable to touch. Gather candy together and, with buttered hands, pull in ropes. Continue to pull until candy gets light in color and hard to pull. Cut candy in half with buttered scissors. Pull each piece into a long strand about half an inch thick. Snip in bite-size pieces and wrap each in wax paper.

Note: If you are sensitive to food colors, try ⅛ tsp. turmeric to color the candy a light yellow.

Molasses taffy: Substitute molasses for the corn syrup, omit salt. Use only ⅓ c. water. Cook to 268° F., then add the Tbsp. margarine and ⅛ tsp. baking soda. Continue as above.

MEAT AND MAIN DISHES

Low-Fat Beef Stroganoff ✓

serves 4

Lower in calories and much lower in fat than the typical stroganoff recipe made with sour cream, this hearty dish is sure to please everyone in the family.

¾ c. "sour cream" base (see recipe, under Miscellaneous)
3 Tbsp. flour
3 Tbsp. water
⅓ c. onion, chopped
2 cloves garlic, minced
1 Tbsp. margarine
1 Tbsp. cooking oil
1 lb. sirloin steak
1¾ c. fat-free beef broth ★
¼ c. cooking sherry
1¼ tsp. dried basil
1¼ tsp. dried marjoram
¼ c. fresh mushrooms or canned, drained mushrooms
salt and pepper to taste
hot, cooked, fettucine noodles

Cut sirloin in thin strips. Combine the "sour cream" base, flour, and water, mixing thoroughly. Set aside.

In skillet over medium heat, saute the onion and garlic in margarine until onion is soft. Remove and set aside. Add cooking oil and fry meat strips until browned. Stir in broth, sherry, basil and marjoram, scraping up the browned bits from bottom of pan. Bring to boil, and add the cooked onion and garlic.

Add about ¼ cup of the hot broth to the "sour cream" base and stir to mix. Then turn heat under skillet to low and pour the "sour cream" mixture back into the skillet gradually, while stirring. Simmer covered until it thickens and flavors blend, about 5 minutes. Serve over hot noodles.

Note: The alcohol in the sherry will boil off.

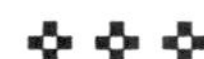

Famous Firehouse Meatloaf

serves 5

1½ lb. lean ground beef
½ c. toasted wheat germ
½ c. unseasoned bread crumbs
3 egg whites
6 Tbsp. lowfat milk
¾ tsp. salt
¾ tsp. garlic powder
¾ tsp. poultry seasoning
½ tsp. dried oregano
½ tsp. dried basil
dash pepper

Preheat oven to 350° F. and spray a loaf pan with non-stick spray or coat with cooking oil. Mix all ingredients thoroughly and pat into a loaf shape in pan. Bake at 350° F. for 1 hour and 20 minutes, or until loaf is done. Let it sit about 10 minutes before slicing.

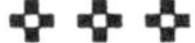

Stuffed Mushroom-Beef Roll

serves 4 to 6

Meat:

⅓ c. beef broth ★

½ c. quick-cooking oats

¼ c. chopped mushrooms (fresh or canned)

2 lbs. very lean ground beef

2 eggs

1 slice whole wheat bread, crumbled

½ tsp. garlic powder

½ tsp. onion salt

dash pepper

Filling:

1 c. chopped mushrooms

2 Tbsp. margarine

½ tsp. dried basil

6 oz. Muenster cheese, thinly sliced (see note)

⅛ tsp. dried oregano

In large bowl combine all of the ingredients for the meat, mixing and kneading very well.

Cover a cookie sheet or wooden board with a large piece of aluminum foil (so cleanup is easy). Wet hands and spread out meat mixture on foil so that it forms a rectangle about 14 inches by 10 inches. (It should be about ¾ of an inch thick). Place whole thing in refrigerator to chill about 20 minutes.

Meanwhile, start making the filling by melting margarine in a saucepan. Add chopped mushrooms, dried basil and oregano. Cook mushrooms over medium heat until most of the moisture is evaporated.

Preheat oven to 350ºF. Remove meat from refrigerator and spread mushroom mixture evenly on meat. Cover mushrooms with slices of cheese, (sliced about ⅛-inch thick). Leave a one inch margin around edge of meat uncovered by cheese, so that filling doesn't ooze out.

Roll up meat, starting at a narrow side. (Lifting foil as you roll helps). When you reach the end, fold down ends of the meat and crimp. Place the roll seam-side down in a 9-inch x 5-inch loaf pan. Bake at 350ºF. for 1 hour and 20 minutes or until meat is done.

Cool for 10 minutes before slicing.

Note: Be sure to cut off the orange rind of the cheese. It could have a high tyramine level and oleoresin paprika, which some are sensitive to.

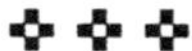

Hawaiian Barbecued Steaks

serves 2

Very little soy sauce remains in the meat, so for those who can have some low-sodium soy sauce, these steaks are a tasty and mouth-watering summer fare.

2 ¾-lb. top sirloin steaks

2 Tbsp. cooking oil

2 Tbsp. pear juice

2 Tbsp. low-sodium soy sauce ★

¼ c. water

½ tsp. ground ginger

½ tsp. garlic powder

¼ tsp. coriander

Pierce steaks with a fork in several places on each side. Combine other ingredients in a shallow covered dish or ziplock bag. Marinate meat overnight. Remove meat from marinade, drain well, and grill over medium hot coals until done.

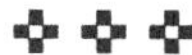

Basil-Braised Beef Roast Dinner ✓

serves 4 or 5

1 2½-lb. beef roast

2 Tbsp. cooking oil

2 or 3 large carrots, peeled and cut in chunks

4 medium boiling potatoes, peeled and quartered

½ tsp. black pepper (optional)

2 tsp. dried basil

¼ tsp. garlic powder

In a heavy skillet, brown roast on all sides in oil. Pierce with a fork on top and sides. Spray baking pan or casserole dish with non-stick cooking spray (or coat with oil). Place roast in baking dish, surrounded by carrots and potatoes.

Add 1 cup water to hot skillet and scrape up crusty bits to make pan juices. Pour the pan juices over meat and potatoes. Sprinkle top of meat with pepper, basil, and garlic powder.

Insert meat thermometer and bake uncovered at 325° F., until temperature of meat is 160° F. (about 1½ to 2 hrs). Once or twice during cooking, turn the potatoes in the meat juices or baste).

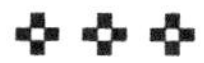

Cheese Topped Mini-Meatloaves ✓

serves 4

1 lb. very lean ground beef

1 large egg

¼ c. shredded raw russet potato

¼ c. chopped onion

¼ c. chopped bell pepper

¼ tsp. allspice

¼ tsp. salt

⅛ tsp. pepper

1 c. Rice Krispie-type cereal

4 slices Muenster or Mozzarella cheese

Coat 8 muffin cups with non-stick cooking spray, margarine, or oil. In bowl, combine all the ingredients except cereal and cheese. Mix well. Add rice cereal last, mixing in just until uniform consistency. Pat into muffin cups, filling to within about ¼ inch of the top. Bake at 400° F. for about 25 minutes. When done, remove loaves from tins and drain on paper towels for a minute or two. Meanwhile, cut cheese in strips about ⅛-inch thick and 1 inch wide. Criss-cross two strips on top of each loaf. (Be sure to remove the orange rind from Muenster, especially if you are sensitive to oleoresin paprika). Place loaves on a heat-proof platter and return to oven just until cheese begins to melt.

Note: This recipe works well as a regular meatloaf too, and is a good loaf for those sensitive to wheat. Check that you use rice cereal that doesn't have the allergenic preservatives BHA or BHT.

Avoiding Nitrates and Nitrites in Meat Products

Nitrate and nitrite compounds have been used for many years to preserve foods, and are considered safe by the Food and Drug Administration. Recently though, safety concerns have been raised because of their link to cancer-causing nitrosamines. Those of us with IC however, have another reason to avoid these additives: they can cause bladder symptom flare-ups.

Partly as a result of public concern over the nitrosamine issue, there are now some resources on the market that may enable some people with IC to eat sausages and such again.

Home sausage making

One way to avoid additives in sausages and other meat products, is to make it yourself. This seems to be the latest culinary fad, and it may also be a boon to IC patients. One of many good books beginning to show up on book-store shelves is *Home Sausage Making* by Charles Reavis (Storey Communications). In his book, Mr. Reavis not only tells how to make your own nitrate-free, MSG-free, sausages and hot dogs, but his recipes are also considerably lower in fat than typical supermarket fare. (Mr. Reavis' recipes have from one-half to one-quarter the fat of similar commercially produced products).

There is another advantage of the make-your-own strategy for IC patients. You can omit the hot spices such as cayenne. (When you make your own, you can also omit what my daughter used to call "the really gross stuff," animal by-products. Manufacturers refer to it as "variety meats").

The sausage-making process isn't difficult, and doesn't take a lot of expensive materials or machinery, but you do have to be very careful about cleanliness. Home sausage making can be fun too, and time-consuming. (Freezing a large batch at temperatures below 0° F. is the best strategy).

If you don't have your grandmother's meat grinder or sausage-stuffing attachment, don't fret. They are both available from the *Chef's Catalog* (3215 Commercial Ave., Northbrook, IL 60062-1900. To order a catalog, call (800) 967-2433). And, if it has anything to do with sausage making, smoking, or meat curing, you can find it in *The Sausage Maker*. This wonderful mail-order catalog lists every kind of smoker, sausage stuffer, or meat grinder available, and you can also order casings (natural or synthetic, from collagen). For a catalog, write: *The Sausage Maker*, 26 Military Road, Buffalo, NY 14207 or call (716) 876-5521.

Buying nitrate-free meat products

You are fortunate if you live in an urban area such as New York or Los Angeles. The multi-ethnic cultures in these areas attract small restaurants and sausage-makers which make meat products to sell locally. You can find excellent quality meat, processed according to old-world family recipes, and often proudly nitrate- and MSG-free. For natural products, don't forget to check the stores listed in Appendix B.

In the area where I live for instance, a family-owned Italian sausage business churns out additive-free Mexican and Italian sausages. They are sold to restaurants under one name but a bit of investigation turned up the fact that they also sell this sausage to a local market under another label. Just finding one sausage product that I could treat myself to now and then, gave me such a sense of freedom and normalcy.

Smoked products

Check your phone book for small businesses that sell gourmet or custom-smoked products. Often they will have some items without additives. The markets listed in Appendix B often sell nitrate-free smoked meat and fish also.

Your local bookstore is a good resource for books with instructions on how to smoke or cure ham, fish, and other meat products cheaply at home.

Before you invest in any costly equipment though, make sure your bladder can tolerate additive-free smoked products. Even without any additives, smoked products can contain high levels of tyramine, a substance suspected of triggering bladder pain for those with IC. (Bacteria which live on the surface of smoked meats, are effective at turning tyrosine, an amino acid found in meat protein, into tyramine).

Pear-Smothered Pork Chops ✓

serves 2

2 center-cut pork loin chops, about ¾" thick

¼ tsp. ground sage

dash salt and pepper

1 large, firm-ripe pear

2 Tbsp. unsulphured molasses

1 Tbsp. flour

1 c. water

In a skillet, brown pork chops in vegetable oil, seasoning with salt and pepper if desired. Remove chops to casserole dish. Sprinkle sage on chops.

Peel and slice pear, placing slices on top of chops. Combine flour with small amount of water to make paste, then add to cup of water. Add molasses to water and mix well. Over low heat, pour liquid into hot skillet, scraping up browned bits of pork chops. When slightly thickened, pour sauce over chops, cover, and bake at 350° F. for 40 minutes, or until done.

Pork Chops with Beans and Bell Pepper

serves 4

2 cloves minced garlic
1 small green bell pepper, seeded
1 small red bell pepper, seeded
vegetable oil
4 pork chops, medium slice
salt and pepper to taste
⅓ c. sherry (see note)
1 tsp. dried thyme
1 1-lb. can Bush's or B&M baked beans
1 1-lb can kidney beans, drained and rinsed
1 c. frozen, sliced carrots or ½ c. canned sliced beets

Preheat oven to 425° F. Cut red and green bell pepper in half-inch chunks. Saute garlic and bell pepper in a little oil about 2 minutes. Remove vegetables and set aside. Season pork chops with salt and pepper if desired, and brown in remaining oil. Add sherry to frying pan and scrape up browned bits. Pour into the resulting hot broth into a 10-inch square casserole dish.

Add bell pepper and garlic, carrots and beans to casserole dish, mixing thoroughly. Top with pork chops. Bake in oven for about 15 minutes, until pork chops are done and beans are bubbly.

Note: Adding wine to hot frying pan boils off the alcohol. Be sure the baked beans don't have a tomato-base sauce.

Italian Baked Chicken ✓

serves 2

2 chicken breast halves, skinless
⅓ c. unseasoned bread crumbs
½ tsp. dried oregano
¼ tsp. dried marjoram
⅛ tsp. salt
⅛ tsp. pepper (see note)
1 egg white, slightly whisked
3 Tbsp. margarine, melted

Rinse and dry chicken. Preheat oven to 375° F. In a bowl, combine bread crumbs with oregano, marjoram, salt and pepper. Roll chicken in egg white, then in the crumb mixture to coat. Pour the melted butter in shallow baking dish and turn chicken pieces in it to coat. Arrange pieces in baking dish (best if they don't touch), and bake at 375° F. until tender, about 50 minutes. Do not turn. Lift out carefully from pan with spatula.

Note: For those who need a low-oxalate version, omit pepper.

Baked Chicken Croquettes

serves 4

4 chicken breasts (boneless, skinless)
2 small, inner stalks of celery with leaves
4 Tbsp. margarine (at room temp.)
4 tsp. grated lemon peel

salt and pepper to taste
1 egg white, slightly beaten
¾ c. unseasoned bread crumbs
3 Tbsp. margarine, melted

Preheat oven to 350° F. Pound chicken breasts until they are about ¼ inch thick. Chop the celery and leaves, making about ¼ cup when chopped. Combine the room temperature margarine with the grated lemon peel and the celery. Spread on each piece of chicken, dividing evenly. Season with salt and pepper. Roll each chicken piece up and secure with a toothpick, then dip or brush with egg white. Coat each piece of chicken in bread crumbs. Pour melted margarine into casserole dish. Roll chicken in melted margarine to coat. Bake, covered, in 350° F. oven for 45 minutes or until chicken is done.

Marinades and Flavorful Meat

Marinades are used not only to enhance the flavor of meat, but also to increase tenderness. It is the acid in marinades that gives them their ability to tenderize. Tough meat or poultry becomes tender as the acid breaks down the meat's stringy fibers. For people with IC though, eating meat drenched in an acidic marinade, may be risking a symptom flare. Worse yet, most commercially prepared marinades contain additives, such as MSG.

You may be able to get away with a homemade, additive-free marinade if you drain the meat well before cooking. Making your own marinade and then draining the meat is not an altogether satisfactory tactic for some people, though, because all marinade recipes use at least some lemon juice, vinegar, or other acid ingredient. For these people even the small amount of acid left in the meat may be too much for their hypersensitive bladders.

Here is an alternative way to give meats flavor and tenderize them that even the most sensitive bladder should tolerate:

✦ First, pierce the meat with a fork or pound it with a meat hammer to break up the fibers and tenderize.

✦ Next, rub the surface with the spices of your favorite marinade recipe. The meat will take up much of the flavor.

✦ Third, be sure to let the spice-rubbed meat sit in the refrigerator for several hours or overnight. This will give the spices time to penetrate the meat.

Besides eliminating the bladder-irritating acidity problem, there is another benefit to this method. When an acid marinade breaks down the meat fiber, the meat loses some of its fluid, becoming drier. The effect of this dehydration is somewhat offset by the absorption of some of the marinade's juice and flavor. Often though, over-marinated meat can become dried out. By rubbing the spices into the meat, and avoiding the acid, your cooked meat may be juicier than if it was marinated in a liquid.

Chinese Five-Spice Chicken ✓

serves 4

This dish is a tasty oriental treat and one of my husband's favorites. It reheats well, so it can be made ahead for parties or potlucks. The soy sauce and onions are discarded so my bladder tolerates it well.

3 Tbsp. soy sauce, low sodium ★
⅓ c. water
1 medium red onion, chopped
1 tsp. powdered ginger
1 clove garlic, minced
1 dash pepper (see note)

4 skinless, boneless, chicken breast halves
1 tsp. cinnamon
½ tsp. allspice
¾ tsp. anise seed
¼ tsp. fennel seed
¼ tsp. powdered ginger

Combine first six of ingredients in a shallow dish or plastic bag and mix well. Pierce chicken once or twice with fork. Add chicken pieces to the marinade and cover dish or seal bag. Refrigerate at least six hours, turning once. Preheat oven to 325° F. Drain chicken pieces and discard the marinade.

Transfer chicken to baking dish that has been lightly oiled, or sprayed with non-stick coating. Combine the last five ingredients in small dish or measuring cup. Sprinkle half the spices over chicken. Cover and bake 325° F. for about 50 minutes. Turn chicken, then sprinkle with remaining spices, and bake uncovered about 10 minutes more, or until tender and fully cooked.

Note: For a low-oxalate version, omit the pepper.

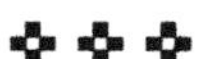

Crispy-Topped Poultry Loaf ✓

serves 4

Meatloaf:
1 lb. extra lean ground beef
1 lb. ground turkey (see note)
1 egg white
6 Tbsp. unseasoned bread crumbs
2 Tbsp. milk
1½ tsp. onion salt
½ tsp. garlic powder
¼ tsp. poultry seasoning

Topping:
20 saltine crackers, crushed
1 egg white, lightly beaten
¼ tsp. poultry seasoning
⅓ c. chicken broth

Preheat oven to 350° F. and lightly spray a 9-inch by 5-inch loaf pan with non-stick cooking spray. In a bowl, combine all the meatloaf ingredients, mixing thoroughly.

Pat the meat into the bottom of the loaf pan. In a bowl, mix together all the ingredients for the topping. Spread the topping mix on the meatloaf, leaving about ¼ inch around the edges, to keep the topping from sticking to the pan. Bake for 1 hour and 10 minutes at 350° F. Let cool for about five minutes before slicing and serving.

Note: Packaged ground turkey can have MSG in it, sometimes referred to on the label as "natural flavoring." I buy turkey breasts and ask someone at the market's meat department to grind it up for me. Ground chicken works well too.

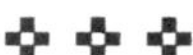

Chicken Cornbread Casserole

serves 3

2 Tbsp. butter or margarine

5 Tbsp. all-purpose flour

1¼ c. low-sodium chicken broth, divided ★

1 c. low-fat milk

1 tsp. onion salt

⅛ tsp. garlic powder

dash pepper, optional

1½ c. cornbread crumbs

½ c. chopped celery

non-stick cooking spray

3 c. cooked chicken, in bite-sized pieces (takes approx. 3 large breast pieces)

2 Tbsp. finely chopped chives, optional

In a medium saucepan melt the margarine. Remove from heat and stir in the flour until it is all absorbed by the butter. Return pan to low heat and stir in 1 cup of the chicken broth, the milk, onion salt, garlic powder, and pepper. Continue to cook and stir until sauce is thickened (don't boil), then set aside.

Preheat oven to 325° F. Combine crumbs and celery in a bowl, pouring remaining ¼ cup chicken broth over crumb mixture, and tossing lightly.

Spray a 10-inch square casserole or baking dish with cooking spray, then place half the chicken pieces on the bottom. Cover with half the crumb mixture. Layer the remaining chicken, then the remaining crumb mixture, and top with the sauce poured over all.

Sprinkle chopped chives on top of sauce. Bake covered at 350° F. until hot and bubbly, about 30 to 35 min. minutes.

Note: This can be made ahead, refrigerated, then popped in the oven at the last minute. If the casserole is cold when you put it in the oven, increase baking time by 5 minutes. This recipe works very well with leftover turkey too.

If you substitute a salty chicken broth for the low-sodium version, omit the onion salt and use ½ tsp. onion powder instead.

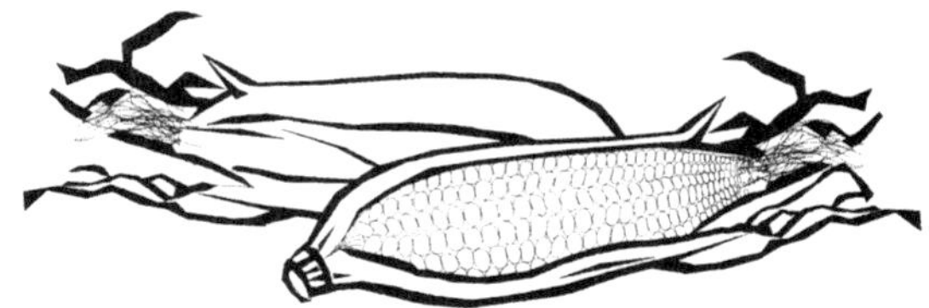

Easy Chicken with Potatoes and Gravy ✓

serves 3

3 boiling potatoes
3 chicken half-breasts, without skin
vegetable oil
1 can Campbell's Healthy Request Mushroom Soup ★
1½ cans water
½ tsp. powdered garlic
½ tsp. ground sage
½ tsp. thyme
salt to taste

Peel or scrub potatoes, halve or cut in large chunks. In large skillet, brown chicken breasts in vegetable oil. Remove chicken. Add mushroom soup, water and spices to hot skillet, stirring to mix thoroughly and break up lumps. Add chicken and potatoes to skillet. Reduce heat, cover and simmer 35 minutes or until chicken is done and potatoes are soft.

Skillet Chicken and Rice Dinner

serves 4

3 Tbsp. margarine, divided
4 chicken thighs, skinned
2 c. sliced fresh mushrooms
½ c. chopped onion
1 c. white rice, uncooked
1½ tsp. dried basil
3 tsp. dried parsley
2 Tbsp. cooking sherry, optional
2 c. chicken broth ★
½ c. water
1 c. frozen green beans
salt and pepper, to taste

Melt 2 Tbsp. of margarine in skillet and brown chicken on all sides. Remove chicken and add remaining margarine. Cook mushrooms and onions, covered, in same pan until soft. Add rice, basil, parsley, sherry, broth, water and green beans. (Alcohol in sherry boils away). Place chicken on top. Cover, reduce heat to simmer, and cook for about 30 minutes. Season with salt and pepper and serve.

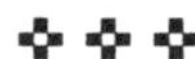

Rosemary Roasted Leg of Lamb

serves 4

3 cloves garlic
1 Tbsp. grated lemon peel
2 Tbsp. dried rosemary, crushed
1 tsp. pepper
1 tsp. salt
½ tsp. dried thyme
½ tsp. ground allspice
pinch of cinnamon
2½ lbs. leg of lamb (boneless)

Mince garlic finely and combine with rest of seasonings in a large ziplock plastic bag. Prick surface of meat all over. Add meat to bag, seal edge securely. Knead meat and seasonings, working the seasonings into the meat. Refrigerate six hours or overnight.

When ready to cook, place meat on rack fatty side up in roasting pan. Add about a cup of water in the bottom of the pan. Insert meat thermometer and cook at 325° F. until meat temperature indicates 175° F., about 1½ to 2 hours.

Let stand about 10 minutes before carving, then slice across grain.

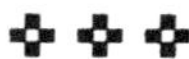

Angie's Vegetarian "Meat"loaf ✿

serves 4

For loaf:

1⅔ c. vegetable broth (or chicken broth)

1 c. lentils

1 Tbsp. finely chopped fresh parsley

½ c. diced onion

⅔ c. diced celery

½ c. finely chopped almonds (or walnuts)

4 slices fresh whole wheat bread, torn

2 saltine crackers, crushed

½ tsp. garlic powder

⅛ tsp. turmeric

½ tsp. poultry seasoning

½ tsp. ground sage

¼ tsp. salt

⅛ tsp. black pepper

3 eggs

2 tsp. molasses

For sauce:

½ c. finely chopped onion

¾ c. finely chopped mushrooms

3 Tbsp. margarine

5 Tbsp. flour

1¾ c. water

Soak lentils in warm water ½ hour. Drain well. In saucepan add lentils to broth and parsley and bring to a boil. Immediately reduce heat to low and simmer covered for 45 minutes. Set aside to cool.

Preheat oven to 350° F. Lightly spray a 9-inch by 5-inch loaf pan with vegetable non-stick cooking spray. In a large bowl mix onion, celery, nuts, bread, crackers, garlic powder, turmeric, poultry seasoning, sage, salt and pepper.

Slightly whisk eggs with molasses and add to vegetables and spices. Drain any remaining broth from lentils and parsley. Combine lentils and other ingredients, kneading to mix well. Place in loaf pan and press down. Bake uncovered at 350° F. for 45 minutes.

Let loaf cool 10 minutes. Meanwhile, make sauce. Melt butter over low heat in a saucepan and add onions. Sauté until onions begin to brown. Add mushrooms, cover, and simmer a couple of minutes until mushrooms are tender. Add flour, stirring to coat. Gradually add water while stirring. When mixture is thick and bubbly, turn loaf out on a serving plate and slice, then pour sauce over slices.

"Dry Marinades" for Grilled Meat

Method for each:

Combine ingredients in a small bowl. Pierce surface of meat if desired. Rub or pound the ingredients into each steak or piece of chicken. Refrigerate in a closed container at least two hours. (You may want to scrape about half the spices off the meat before grilling).

✦ Basic Spices

for 3 beef steaks

2 tsp. black pepper
1½ tsp. onion salt
1 tsp. brown sugar
¼ tsp. garlic powder

✦ Indonesian-style ✓

for 2 beef steaks

1½ tsp. onion salt
½ tsp. finely minced garlic
½ tsp. cinnamon
½ tsp. coriander
¼ tsp. thyme
½ tsp. ginger
2 tsp. sugar

✦ Oriental Blend ✓

for 3 chicken breasts

1 clove garlic, minced
½ c. green onion, chopped
2 tsp. vegetable oil
3 Tbsp. chopped fresh mint leaves
1 tsp. coriander
1 tsp. anise seed
¼ tsp. powdered ginger

Mushroom Frittata ✿

serves 4

4 eggs
4 egg whites
¼ c. milk
1 tsp. dried basil
1 tsp. dried oregano
1 tsp. dried thyme
1 tsp. onion salt
1⅔ c. seeded, diced bell pepper
1½ c. chopped fresh mushrooms
2 oz. mozzarella cheese, shredded

In bowl, beat first seven ingredients until frothy, about 2 minutes.

Preheat oven to 350° F. Coat a very clean skillet with cooking spray or oil and heat over medium heat. Add egg mixture, using a spatula to loosen edges of egg and allow runny part to flow to bottom of pan, as you would with an omelette. Cook until egg is mostly cooked but still a little runny on top. Add mushrooms and bell pepper to top of egg.

Remove frittata and slide carefully into a large casserole dish or other heat-proof dish which has been coated with cooking spray. Sprinkle shredded cheese on top of frittata. Place in oven for 5 minutes, or until egg is set and cheese is melted. To serve, cut in quarters with a knife or a pizza cutter.

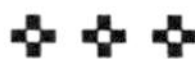

PIES AND DESSERTS

Coconut Cream Pie ✿✓

serves 8

Pie Crust:

1¼ c. flour

½ tsp. salt

⅓ c. margarine (stick, not tub)

3 or 4 Tbsp. water

Filling:

4 egg yolks

1 c. sugar

½ c. flour

¼ tsp. salt

3 c. milk (2% low-fat ok)

2 tsp. vanilla extract

3 Tbsp. butter

1 c. unsweetened shredded coconut ★

Meringue:

4 egg whites

⅛ tsp. cream of tartar

½ c. sugar

¾ tsp. vanilla extract

¼ c. unsweetened shredded coconut ★

To make crust:

Stir together flour and salt. Cut in margarine until texture is like cornmeal. Add water, knead, and form dough into a ball. On lightly floured surface, roll out dough from center to edge, forming circle about 12 inches in diameter. Lay in pie pan, flute edges. Prick sides and bottom with a fork and bake at 450° F. for 10 to 12 minutes, just until slightly golden.

To make filling:

Separate yolks from whites of eggs. Beat egg yolks slightly in small bowl. set aside. In saucepan combine sugar, flour and salt. Stir in milk and cook until thickened and bubbly. Reduce heat and cook, stirring for 2 more minutes. Stir about ½ cup of the hot mixture into the egg yolks. Pour the yolk mixture back into the saucepan and bring to a boil, stirring. Cook 2 minutes more, then remove from heat. Stir in vanilla, butter, and coconut, and pour hot mixture into a cooled, baked pie shell. Let filling cool before making the topping.

To make topping:

Beat egg whites with cream of tartar until soft peaks form. Gradually add sugar and vanilla while beating. Continue to beat until stiff peaks form. Spread meringue over hot pie filling, sealing it to the edge of pie crust. Sprinkle with coconut and bake at 350° F. for 10 to 12 minutes until meringue is golden brown and coconut is toasted.

You can also omit the meringue and, just before serving, scoop a dollop of whipped cream on each piece. If you do this, refrigerate the pie and cover with a plastic wrap to keep the filling from drying out before serving time. *Calories per serving: 479*

Note: Be sure to get coconut that has not been treated with sodium meta-bisulfite. The sulfite may cause bladder symptoms in some people. See the list in Appendix B, for sources of sulfite-free coconut.

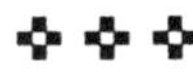

Two-Crust Blueberry Pie ✿

serves 8

¾ c. sugar

3½ Tbsp. flour

½ tsp. nutmeg

dash cinnamon

dash salt

3 c. ripe blueberries

¼ tsp. lemon extract

pastry for 9-inch double crust pie

Preheat oven to 400° F. Combine sugar with flour, nutmeg, cinnamon, and salt. Mix very well. Add blueberries. Stir gently to coat berries until they are evenly coated. Sprinkle with lemon extract. Turn into pastry-lined pie plate. Cover with top crust, cutting several one-inch slits to let steam escape. Brush top crust with milk and sprinkle lightly with sugar. Cover edges with aluminum foil.

Bake at 400° F. for 20 minutes. Remove foil and brush top crust with milk. Sprinkle lightly with sugar. Bake another 20 to 25 minutes until top is golden. *Calories per serving: 366*

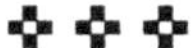

Almond Pear Pie ✿✓

serves 8

To make crust:

2 c. all-purpose flour

1 tsp. salt

⅔ c. margarine, softened (stick kind)

¼ c. finely ground almonds

5 to 7 Tbsp. water

To make filling:

½ c. sugar

¼ tsp. nutmeg

2 Tbsp. all-purpose flour

4 large, firm, pears (not overly ripe)

¼ tsp. almond extract

¼ c. blanched, slivered almonds

¼ c. raisins, dried currants, or chopped dates ★

Mix flour and salt for crust. Cut in margarine until it has an even, crumbly consistency like cornmeal. Add ground almonds, mixing well. Add water until moistened and form into a ball. Divide dough in half. Roll out half of the dough and place in a 9-inch pie pan. Cover with damp cloth until fruit filling is ready.

Preheat oven to 400° F. For filling, mix together the sugar, nutmeg and flour in a large bowl. Peel and slice pears into the bowl, stirring gently to coat. Stir in almond extract, almonds, dried fruit, then turn the mixture into pie crust. Roll out top pie crust layer, and place on top of fruit, sealing edges. Cut slits in top crust, and bake at 400° F. for 55 minutes. Cover the crust edge with aluminum foil for the first 15 minutes to keep it from burning. *Calories per serving: 420*

Note: If omitting dried fruit in the filling, increase almonds to ½ cup and flour to 3 Tbsp.

Pear Crumble Pie 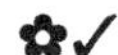

serves 8

Pastry for 9-inch single crust pie

For Filling:

⅓ c. sugar

½ tsp. cornstarch

2 Tbsp. flour

⅛ tsp. cinnamon

5 c. sliced, peeled, firm pears

For Topping:

⅓ c. sugar

⅔ c. flour

½ tsp. cinnamon

¼ tsp. ginger

⅓ c. butter or margarine, softened

Roll out pastry and line a 9-inch pie plate. Trim and flute the edge.

Preheat oven to 400° F. In a bowl mix together thoroughly the sugar, cornstarch, flour and cinnamon for the filling. Slice pears and toss with the flour mixture to coat.

In another bowl, combine the sugar, flour and spices for the topping. Cut in the butter until crumbly, and lumps are the size of peas. Turn pears into the pastry-lined plate and sprinkle topping over the pie. Bake in 400° F. oven until topping is a golden brown, about 45 minutes. Covering the edges with foil for the first 30 minutes of baking helps keep the edges from burning. *Calories per serving: 240*

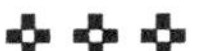

Pie Dress-Ups

Pastry chefs at famous restaurants can make a plain-Jane pie look elegant with a few simple tricks. Here are some ways to make any pie more appetizing or glamorous:

✦ Make a cut-out edge for a single-crust pie

Make a little more pastry than usual for a single crust pie. Roll out the pastry for the pie crust and lay in the pan. Trim the edge of the pastry even with the edge of the pie plate. (Cover the pastry to keep it from drying out while you do the next step). Roll out the remaining dough quite thin and use hors d'oeuvre cutters or a knife to cut small shapes such as leaves or flowers out of the dough. Brush the edge of the pastry with water and gently press the shapes onto the edge, overlapping each slightly and working your way around the pie. Fill and bake as directed in the recipe.

✦ Put cut-out pastry shapes on a custard-type pie

Make a little extra pastry and roll it out thin. Cut out shapes with a cookie cutter, a knife, or an hors d'oeuvre cutter. Place the cut-outs on a cookie sheet and bake at 400° F. for about 5 minutes, or until golden brown. (Watch carefully, they burn easily!) Cool on the cookie sheet, then remove and set aside. Later, place them on top of the cooled pie filling.

✦ Give it some cheerful color

Sprinkle multi-color cake decors on the top of a meringue pie before baking the meringue. (Don't use colored sugar crystals, they may melt in the meringue).

Tinted coconut or chopped nuts can also give a meringue top an interesting look.

✦ **Make an evenly browned crust**

Lightly brush the top of a double- crust pie with milk. (Don't use so much that it puddles. Regular milk works better than low-fat). Bake as directed in the recipe.

✦ **Make a shiny crust**

Beat an egg white slightly. Brush on the crust just before baking.

✦ **Make a pie top glisten with sugar crystals**

Sprinkle a light coating of sugar evenly over the top of the pie crust after brushing it with cream or milk. Then bake as directed.

Pumpkin Chiffon Tart ✿✓

serves 8

For Pastry:

2 c. flour
½ tsp. sugar
¼ tsp. salt
½ c. unsalted butter, melted
¼ c. unsalted butter (very cold)
1 Tbsp. finely chopped almonds
¼ c. cold water

For Filling:

1 envelope unflavored gelatin
½ c. sugar
½ tsp. salt
¾ tsp. allspice
¼ tsp. powdered ginger
2 tsp. grated orange peel
1 c. canned pumpkin
¾ c. milk
2 egg yolks
2 egg whites
¼ c. sugar
½ c. whipping cream

Sift together the flour, sugar, and salt for the pastry. Add melted butter and cut in with a pastry blender until it has texture of peas or oatmeal.

Preheat oven to 375° F. Cut the cold butter in cubes, about ½-inch square. Add butter cubes to the flour mixture. Toss to coat cubes with mixture. Add cold water and almonds. Knead until malleable, but leave little bits of plain butter. (The volume of water is approximate; adjust it by the dough's consistency).

Gently roll out the dough to a ¼-inch thickness and lay in a 10-inch tart pan. Trim the edges to the top of the tart pan, and prick bottom of pastry with a fork. Bake in oven at 375° F. for about ten minutes or until golden brown. Chill tart shell.

In a saucepan, thoroughly mix gelatin, sugar, salt, allspice and ginger for the filling. Stir in peel, pumpkin, milk and egg yolks. Cook over medium heat, stirring, just to boiling. Set in the regrigerator and chill until it begins to set, about 15 minutes. Meanwhile, beat the egg whites until soft peaks form. Gradually add ¼ cup sugar while continuing to beat until stiff peaks form. Whip the cream until soft peaks form. Gently fold the egg whites and whipped cream into pumpkin. Spoon into tart shell. Chill until firm. *Calories per serving: 486*

Blueberry-Cream Cheese Tart ✿

serves 8

For Pastry:

2 c. all-purpose flour

½ tsp. sugar

¼ tsp. salt

¼ c. unsalted butter, melted

½ c. unsalted butter, refrigerated

¼ c. cold water

For Filling:

12 oz. cream cheese, softened

1 tsp. vanilla extract

½ c. sugar

½ c. whipping cream

2 to 2½ c. fresh blueberries

For Glaze:

2½ c. fresh blueberries

¾ c. sugar

2 Tbsp. cornstarch

¼ tsp. nutmeg

¼ tsp. baking soda

2 tsp. water

Sift together the flour, sugar, and salt for tart shell. Add melted butter and cut in with a pastry blender until texture of cornmeal. Cut cold butter in cubes, about ½-inch square. Add butter cubes to the flour mixture and toss to coat cubes. Add cold water and knead until pliable, but leave little bits of plain butter.

Preheat oven to 375° F. Gently roll out the dough on a floured surface. Roll to ¼-inch thickness and lay in a non-stick tart pan (or one coated with non-stick cooking spray). Trim the edges even with top of tart pan and prick bottom of pastry with a fork. Bake at 375° F. for about 12 minutes until lightly browned. Let cool in pan 10 minutes, then remove pastry, place on serving plate, and chill in refrigerator.

While tart shell is chilling, make filling. With a mixer, beat cream cheese with vanilla and sugar until fluffy, then set aside. Whip whipping cream until stiff peaks form. Gently fold whipped cream into cream cheese mixture.

Remove chilled tart shell from refrigerator and fill with cream cheese mixture. Cover top of cream cheese with the blueberries reserved for filling. Return to refrigerator for 20 minutes.

Meanwhile, make glaze. In a small saucepan mix together sugar and cornstarch for the glaze. Add nutmeg, baking soda, water, and blueberries reserved for the glaze. Cook over medium heat while stirring, until mixture comes to a rolling boil and liquid is slightly thickened. Mash berries and continue cooking until it is a deep purple and there is no foam. Remove from heat and pour through a sieve to remove berry skins. Spread glaze over blueberries with spatula, forcing it between berries. Chill tart at least 1 hour before serving. *Calories per serving: 651*

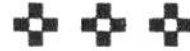

Blueberry Benefits

One fruit that most people with IC seem to tolerate well is the blueberry. Botanical cousin of the cranberry, it is free of the cranberry's sharp acidity. It's very tasty, mild, and sweet when ripe, and may have some health benefits, too. The School of Public Health at the University of California, Berkeley, reports that many fruits and vegetables are high in antioxidant vitamins such as vitamins C and E. (An antioxidant is a substance that can deactivate the free radicals that damage cells and promote heart disease or cancer). Besides having vitamins C and E, fruits and vegetables also have other compounds that act as antioxidants. In a test-tube study which compared the ability of dozens of fruits and vegetables to mop up free radicals, blueberries ranked first. Other "IC safe" foods such as broccoli, corn, and pears also had impressive abilities to neutralize free radicals.

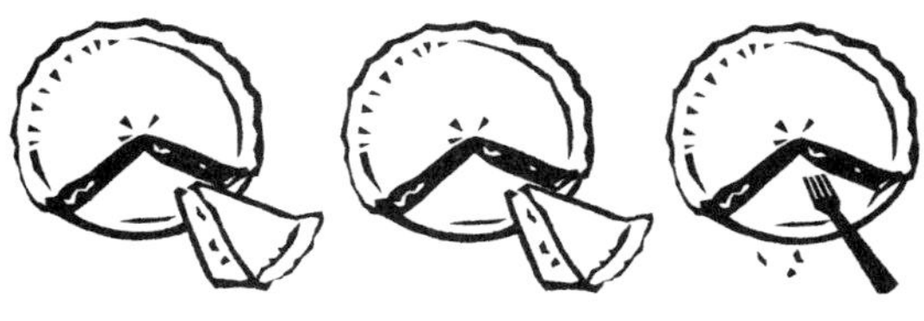

Blueberry Fool ✿

serves 3

This is a frothy and elegant dessert to serve for get-togethers with friends or romantic candlelight dinners.

¾ cup lowfat milk
6 oz. fresh blueberries (about 1 cup)
2 Tbsp. water
2 Tbsp. sugar
⅛ tsp. mace
¼ tsp. cinnamon

2 Tbsp. flour
2 Tbsp sugar
3 egg yolks
1 tsp. vanilla
½ c. heavy whipping cream
whipped cream, blanched almonds, mint sprigs, for decoration (optional)

Refrigerate a large bowl to get it cold. In a small saucepan, bring milk to a boil. Remove milk from heat and set aside to cool.

Meanwhile, put blueberries in another saucepan with the water, cover and simmer over medium heat until soft, about six minutes. Remove from heat and add sugar, mace, and cinnamon to berries. Pour into a shallow pan (like a pie pan). Set pan of berries in freezer.

While berries are cooling, in a clean saucepan combine the flour and 2 Tbsp. sugar. Whisk in egg yolks. Whisk in the scalded milk until the ingredients are thoroughly combined. Cook over low heat, stirring constantly until the mixture thickens, about 2 or 3 minutes. Continue to simmer and stir over very low heat until it is the consistency of pudding. Stir in the vanilla, and set aside to cool.

Bring chilled bowl from refrigerator and pour in whipping cream. Whip until stiff peaks form. Set back in refrigerator for a moment. Fold the cold blueberries into the thickened yolk mixture. Re- move whipped cream from the refrig- erator and fold that in as well. Spoon into stemmed glasses (add to the center of the glass to keep the rim clean). Chill 2 hours before serving. *Calories per serving: 414*

To decorate, if desired:

Nut topping — Heat 2 tsp. vegetable oil in a skillet over medium heat. When hot, add slivered, blanched almonds. Heat, stirring until nuts start to brown. Remove and blot excess oil with paper towel. When cool, chop in a food processor or by hand. Chill the chopped nuts. At serving time, spoon whipped cream on top of chilled desserts, then sprinkle nuts on the center of each. (Make sure nuts are cooled, or they may melt the whipped cream).

Mint topping— Spoon a dollop of whipped cream in the center of each dessert. Stick a small sprig of mint on the whipped cream.

To use other fruit :

If you can tolerate raspberries or blackberries, this recipe works very well with them too, when the acidity is partially neutralized. For raspberries: eliminate the mace and cinnamon, and add an additional tablespoon of sugar, as well as a quarter teaspoon of baking soda, to the berries after cooking. For blackberries: cook in water, then sieve out the seeds. Omit the mace and cinnamon, and add an extra tablespoon of sugar and a pinch of baking soda to cooked berries.

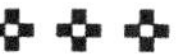

Sichuan Baked Pears 

serves 2

Fragrant and sweet, glazed pears make a wonderful light dessert after a meal. Although in China they wouldn't think of serving the warm pears with vanilla ice cream on the side, it's a wonderful treat that way).

1½ Tbsp. butter
2 firm pears, peeled
3 Tbsp. sugar
⅛ tsp. cinnamon
⅛ tsp. anise seed
⅛ tsp. allspice
⅛ tsp. coriander

Preheat oven to 400° F. Melt butter and pour into a shallow baking dish. Core pears and cut in quarters. Place in butter, turning to coat. Mix sugar and spices and sprinkle over pears. Bake at 400° F. for 5 minutes. Baste with pan juices. Bake another 7 minutes until sugar is bubbly. Cool slightly, then serve warm. *Calories per serving: 247*

Cloves and Cinnamon

Along with black pepper and cinnamon, cloves are one of the most popular and widely used seasonings. Imported from Malaysia and the island of Madagascar, cloves are dried flower buds of the clove tree. As the buds swell and mature, an oily aromatic substance called eugenol develops. Eugenol, sometimes called eugenic acid, gives cloves their pungent aroma and is responsible for flavoring foods cooked with cloves. In the stomach, eugenol promotes the secretion of gastric acid. For IC patients, cloves may cause flare-ups of bladder symptoms. Allspice and cinnamon also contain eugenol, but in much smaller quantities. Many IC patients have no problems with allspice or cinnamon. In some recipes, these spices can replace cloves. Watch out though, for commercially-baked products containing a type of cinnamon which is promoted as very strong and intensely flavorful. This pungent cinnamon may trigger an increase in bladder pain and frequency.

Wheat-Free Blackberry Soufflé ✿

serves 4

1 Tbsp. butter
2 Tbsp. sugar
½ tsp. vanilla
6 oz. ripe blackberries, fresh or thawed frozen (see note)
2 egg whites
¼ c. sugar
whipped cream

Coat four half-cup custard dishes, individual soufflé dishes, or ramekins with butter. Preheat the oven to 350° F. In a blender or food processor, puree the blackberries, then strain out seeds. Stir 2 Tbsp. sugar and the vanilla into puree, mixing thoroughly.

Beat egg whites until soft peaks form, then add ¼ c. sugar and continue beating until stiff peaks form. Fold in blackberry puree. Fill soufflé dishes and bake at 350° F. for 10 minutes. (Top of soufflés will be above top of dishes by about half the depth of the dishes). Let cool for 15 minutes, then refrigerate for 1 hour. Top with whipped cream just before serving. *Calories per serving: 129*

Note: This recipe balances the acid in the blackberries with the alkalinity of egg white. Egg white will neutralize the fruit acid sufficiently for me, but if you find it still is too acid, try adding a pinch of baking powder to the blackberry puree.

Quick Desserts ✿✓

Here are some ideas to make elegant-looking, but IC-friendly, desserts when you're in a hurry:

✦ Top a custard dish full of fresh, chilled, blueberries with whipped cream and a sprig of mint.

✦ Cut watermelon and honeydew melon in half-inch cubes. Layer the melon cubes in a stemmed glass, giving a green and pink striped effect. Top with a spoonful of whipped cream, sprinkled with a dash of ground coriander. (Use only honeydew if watermelon is too acid for you).

✦ Layer small cubes of pound cake, home made blueberry dessert topping (canned pie filling is easier if your body can tolerate it), and whipped cream, in a dessert dish.

✦ Roll a scoop of all-natural vanilla ice cream in any chopped nuts your body can tolerate, and return to freezer for an hour or so to re-set firm before serving. Kids enjoy ice cream scoops rolled in cake decors or crushed peppermint candies!

✦ And speaking of kids...they love to eat "spaghetti" for dessert. Press vanilla ice cream or frozen yogurt through a potato ricer to make "spaghetti." Top with some raspberry preserves for the "sauce" and raisins for the "meatballs."

Homemade Berry Dessert Topping ✿

Ice cream, cheesecakes, and pound cakes can all be dressed up with a little dessert topping. This delicious topping keeps for quite awhile in the refrigerator and has none of the citric acid or artificial ingredients that purchased toppings can have.

½ c. sugar
2 Tbsp. flour
¼ tsp. ground cinnamon
2 c. fresh, ripe blueberries or blackberries
¼ tsp. lemon extract
¼ c. water

Thoroughly mix the sugar, flour, and cinnamon in a saucepan. Add the blueberries, lemon extract and water. Heat while stirring, coating the blueberries with the sugar. Bring to a rolling boil over medium to high heat, stirring continuously to prevent any scorching. Continue stirring and cooking one minute more. Pour into a heat-proof container to cool. Store in refrigerator until ready to use.

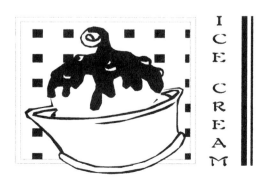

Favorite Cheesecake ✿

serves 12

2 c. graham cracker crumbs ★
⅓ c. finely chopped almonds
⅛ tsp. ground cinnamon
¼ c. butter
¼ c. margarine
3 eggs
2 8-oz. pkgs. cream cheese, softened
¼ tsp. salt
2¼ tsp. vanilla extract
¼ tsp. almond extract
1 c. sugar
1 16-oz. carton low-fat cottage cheese

Mix together the crumbs, almonds and cinnamon. Melt the butter and margarine together and mix with the crumbs. Press on the bottom and sides of a 9-inch springform pan. Beat smooth the eggs, cream cheese, salt, vanilla, almond extract, and sugar. Empty the cottage cheese into a food processor or blender and process until relatively smooth. Beat into the cream cheese mixture. Pour into crust. Bake at 375° F. for 40 min., until just set (filling will be soft). *Calories per serving: 393*

Note: This even more sumptuous served with Homemade Berry Dessert Topping (previous page) or Pears in Cinnamon Syrup (page 77).

Pear variation: Prepare as above but reduce cottage cheese to 8 ounces, and beat in 1 Tbsp. flour with the cream cheese. Chop a peeled, cored pear in half-inch chunks, to make 1 cup. Place pears in boiling water, reduce heat, and simmer 2 minutes. Remove, rinse under cold water and drain well. Stir drained pears into batter and bake at 375° F. for 45 minutes.

Carob chip variation: Prepare batter as usual, stirring in ¼ cup of carob chips. (See Appendix B for sources of chips).

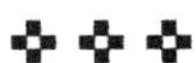

Butterscotch-Pear Tarts ✿✓

makes 4 4-inch or 5-inch tarts

for crust:
1½ c. all-purpose flour
½ tsp. salt
½ c. margarine, at room temperature
5 Tbsp. cold water

for custard filling:
¾ c. brown sugar
3 Tbsp. cornstarch
¼ tsp. salt
2 c. milk
3 egg yolks
3 Tbsp. margarine
1¼ tsp. vanilla extract

for pear topping:
2 Tbsp. light brown sugar
6 Tbsp. sugar
2 tsp. cornstarch
pinch ground cinnamon
5 Tbsp. margarine
4 pears, cored and peeled
whipped cream

Preheat oven to 425° F. Mix together the flour and salt for the crust. Cut in margarine until like small peas. Add cold water and stir just until all is moistened. Divide dough in quarters. Press each piece of dough into a 4-inch or 5-inch individual tart pan with removable bottom. Press dough out so that bottom is about ⅛-inch thick, and sides are about ¼-inch thick. Let sides extend up about half an inch above sides of the pan. Flute as you would a pie crust edge, and prick bottom and sides with a fork. Bake at 425° F. for 12 to 15 minutes, until golden brown. Remove and let cool while making custard.

In a saucepan, thoroughly mix together the brown sugar, cornstarch and salt. Stir in the milk until brown sugar is completely dissolved and mixture is lump-free. Cook over medium heat while stirring, until mixture is bubbly. Continue cooking and stirring for 2 more minutes.

Remove from heat and take out 1 or 2 Tbsp. of hot mixture. Stir the small amount of hot mixture into the egg yolks until blended. Pour egg yolks back into the hot mixture, stir, and place over medium heat again. Cook and stir another 2 minutes.

Remove from heat and stir in margarine and vanilla. Remove tart shells from pans and place on serving plates. Pour custard into tart shells, filling to within ¼-inch of the top. Set tarts aside to cool while making the pear topping.

In saucepan, thoroughly combine the light brown sugar, sugar, cornstarch, and cinnamon. Cut pears in pie-slices. Add margarine to saucepan and cook over medium heat while stirring. Bring to boiling. Add pear slices and continue boiling and stirring until pears are softened and cooked through. Spoon pears over tops of tarts. (There may be a little syrup left over). Chill in the refrigerator at least 2 hours. Top with whipped cream before serving. *Calories per serving: 924*

Banana tart variation: If your bladder is comfortable with bananas, this is a tasty variation. Make tart shells as above. Slice one or two firm-ripe bananas into the shells. Make custard as above but use ½ cup sugar and ¼ cup light brown sugar instead of ¾ cup brown sugar. Pour the custard over the bananas. Chill two hours, top with whipped cream before serving.

Maple-Coconut tarts: The sweet flavor will remind you of pecan pie. Make crust as above, but don't prick with a fork, and don't bake. Thoroughly combine in a bowl: 2 whole eggs (slightly beaten), ⅔ c. sugar, 1 Tbsp. real maple syrup, 4 Tbsp. margarine (melted), 1¼ c. unsweetened shredded coconut ★, and ½ tsp. vanilla. Pour into tart shells and bake at 350° F. for 40 minutes, until filling is set in center. Remove, chill for 2 hours in refrigerator.

Serve topped with whipped cream or decorate: while tart chills in refrigerator, make another recipe of the tart shell dough. Roll out dough to a thickness slightly less than ¼-inch thick on a lightly floured board. Cut four maple-leaf shapes with cookie cutters, tracing "veins" in each with a knife tip. (Or trace a real leaf on heavy paper, and cut the shape out. With a knife, cut dough using the paper shape as a guide). Bake leaf shapes on a cookie sheet at 425° F. about 5 to 10 minutes, just until golden brown. Top each tart with a pastry "maple leaf."

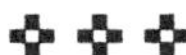

Sherried Pear-Nut Desserts ✿✓

serves 4

½ c. sherry
½ c. sugar
½ c. almonds, sliced
4 pears. peeled, cored and pie-sliced
pinch ginger
½ tsp. cinnamon
4 tsp. cornstarch
4 tsp. water
4 baked Pepperidge Farm pastry shells
vanilla or almond praline ice cream (optional)

In a small saucepan, combine sugar and sherry. Over medium heat, bring to boiling and cook uncovered about one minute (this lets the alcohol evaporate).

Stir in almonds, pear slices, ginger and cinnamon. Cover, reduce heat a bit and simmer 5 minutes.

In a small dish, mix cornstarch and water. Remove two tablespoons of the hot pear liquid and stir into the cornstarch. Pour the cornstarch mixture back into the pears and stir until slightly thickened, about a minute. Remove from heat and let cool about 3 minutes. (Can be made ahead to this point and reheated). To serve, arrange baked pastry shells on plates. Divide warm pears among dessert cups, pouring sauce over each, and letting a little sauce run down the sides. Place a scoop of ice cream on the side of each dessert and top with more sliced almonds. *Calories per serving: 575*

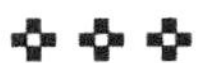

Unusual Pastry Cutters

Although we tend to think of them as "cookie cutters," those whimsical bent-metal shapes can be used creatively with many kinds of foods. They can create appealing heart-shaped biscuits on Valentine's Day, or jazz up Fourth of July burger patties with star-shaped slices of American cheese. Cut-out pastry shapes are especially good for making interesting tops on baked goods (see *Pie Dress-Ups* on page 135). Here is a source of unusual and interesting cutters. They carry the maple-leaf designs used for the Maple-Coconut tarts (page 143). Send a self-addressed stamped envelope and a dollar for a list of their products and an order form.

The Little Fox Factory
931 Marion Road
Bucyrus, OH 44820

SEAFOOD

Salmon in Garlic Basil Sauce ✓

serves 2

2 salmon steaks
¼ c. olive oil
3 cloves fresh garlic, sliced
1 tsp. ground fennel seed
1 tsp. lemon extract (optional)
1 tsp. dried basil
salt and pepper to taste

Combine all ingredients except fish in a food processor or blender and process about 20 seconds. Place fish in a shallow greased baking dish and pour sauce over fish. Cover and bake at 350° F. for 25 minutes or until fish flakes easily with a fork.

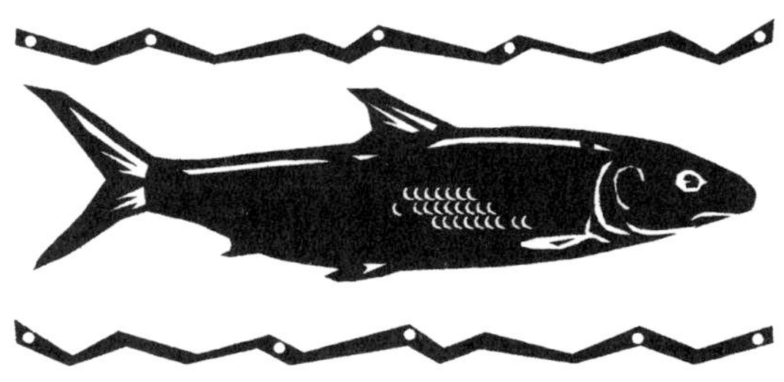

Puget Sound Baked Salmon Steaks

serves 4

3 Tbsp. olive oil
4 salmon steaks (about ½ lb. each)
1½ Tbsp. freshly grated lemon peel
3 Tbsp. brown sugar
¼ tsp. pepper
dash salt, optional

Brush casserole dish and both sides of salmon steaks with olive oil. Sprinkle lemon peel on fish. Top with brown sugar, salt and pepper. Bake in 375° F. oven for 30 min, or till fish flakes easily.

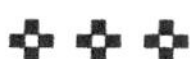

Pacific Ginger-Grilled Salmon ✓

serves 2

1½ lb. salmon fillet, cut in two pieces
2 Tbsp. butter, melted
¼ tsp. salt
¼ tsp. lemon extract (optional)
1 Tbsp. finely minced fresh ginger
dash pepper, optional

Rinse salmon fillet and dry, cut in two pieces. Meanwhile prepare barbecue fire. Set grill about 3 inches above fire. (Two or three moistened, drained wood chips on the coals provide just a light hint of smoke without being overpowering, if you don't have a wood fire).

Mix salt, pepper, lemon extract, melted butter and ginger in small bowl. Place fish on a sheet of heavy-duty aluminum foil. Brush fish with ginger sauce and place the aluminum foil with fish on the grill. Cover and cook salmon about 5-7 minutes. Pour remaining sauce over salmon and cook until opaque through (done), another 7 or 8 minutes. Remove skin before serving, if desired.

Seafood Chowder

serves 3

1 lb. cod or haddock fillets
2 Tbsp. margarine or butter
⅓ c. chopped onion
⅓ c. celery, chopped fine
1 clove garlic, sliced
1½ c. water
1 6-oz. can minced clams
½ tsp. salt
¼ tsp. pepper
⅔ c. white rose potatoes, peeled, cut in one-inch cubes
2 tsp. dried parsley
¼ tsp. dried thyme

1 Tbsp. margarine
¼ c. flour
1¾ c. milk

Cut up fish into cubes, about one inch in size. Melt 2 Tbsp. butter in a large saucepan and cook onion, celery and garlic until soft and slightly golden. Add fish to onions and pour in water. Cover and simmer gently about two minutes. Add clams, salt, pepper, potatoes, parsley, and thyme. Cover and simmer gently about 15 minutes more. Meanwhile, melt another tablespoon of margarine and add flour, mixing well with a fork. Blend the milk gradually into margarine. Turn off heat under the chowder and stir in milk and flour mixture. When combined, turn up heat again and heat through (don't boil), stirring to thicken. Serve.

Scallops Napoli

serves 2

2 Tbsp. butter or margarine
½ tsp. fennel seeds
¼ c. water
1 large bell pepper, cut in thin strips
1 lb. scallops
¼ tsp. onion salt
½ tsp. garlic powder
½ tsp. cornstarch
3 Tbsp. water

Rinse scallops and set aside. Melt butter in skillet. Add fennel seeds, smashing with back of spoon. Add the ¼ cup water and cook over medium heat about 3 minutes. Scrape fennel seeds to one side of skillet and tilt skillet so liquid flows to the other. Remove seeds with spoon or spatula. Add bell pepper to skillet, cover and cook over medium to low heat until tender. Add scallops and cook covered about two minutes.

Combine onion salt, garlic powder, and cornstarch in a small dish. Stir in 3 Tbsp. water. Pour into skillet and cook, stirring scallops until sauce is thick, another minute or two. (Good served with garlic bread and sliced melon).

Buying Fish and Other Seafood

Seafood is a healthy source of protein that many cholesterol-conscious Americans are increasingly turning to. Most seafood is naturally low in cholesterol, and the fat it contains is mainly the health-promoting polyunsaturated kind.

Dr. Joyce Nettleton, a nutritionist, author, and expert on seafood, says the health benefits of eating seafood are just beginning to be explored. One important attribute of fish, she says, is that it's an excellent source of Omega-3 fatty acids. Omega-3 fatty acids are thought to reduce triglycerides in the blood, a factor associated with heart disease. New research by Dr. Joseph Hibbeln, a psychiatrist at the National Institute of Alcohol Abuse and Alcoholism, suggests that omega-3 fatty acids in the diet may also decrease the risk of depression.

Dr. Barry Sears, a biochemist and expert in dietary regulation of hormonal response, notes that, at least in animal research, eating fish oil seems to be effective in fighting cancer. What may be more immediately important to IC patients is that fish contains eicosapentanoic acid (EPA). According to Dr. Sears, EPA is a building block of some substances in the body that act to suppress painful inflammation.

Fish versus fish oil supplements

Doctors and dietary experts often point out the benefits of eating seafood. Although taking fish oil dietary supplements has become popular, simply eating more seafood may be a better bet. Fish gives you protein, and some important nutrients that fish oil capsules don't have.

Dr. Sears also points out that there is no industry regulation requiring the fish oil in dietary supplements to be subjected to molecular distillation, a process that removes heavy metals and pesticides. Fish from polluted waters accumulate such substances in their tissues, and consumers have no way of knowing where the fish oil originated.

Fish quality

When you go to the store to select some fish for dinner, do you really know what they mean by "fresh" fish? In talking to a fisherman and seafood vendor, I was surprised to learn that the word merely means that the fish has not been previously frozen. The word "fresh" as used by supermarkets, implies nothing as to the age or the quality of the fish.

"Fresh-frozen" seafood, however, is often of much better quality than that labelled "fresh." "Fresh-frozen" means that the fish is frozen right on the ship, or at a processing plant on shore, within hours of being caught.

Whatever they call it, when you buy fish at the store it shouldn't have a strong "fishy" odor. If it does, chances are it's old.

Chemical additives in seafood

Sulfites, which are sometimes used by restaurants to keep the greens at salad bars fresh, are also used by seafood processors to inhibit deterioration. A dilute sulfite solution is sometimes used to coat shrimp because certain species will develop unappetizing black spots when exposed to the air for an extended period. Many people are very sensitive to these chemicals and will have allergic reactions. People with IC may have an increase of bladder pain when they eat seafood or other products that have been treated with sulfites.

Fish too, may be treated. It is sometimes dipped in a phosphate solution to keep it from spoiling. Although phosphates haven't been proven harmful to humans, if the solution is too concentrated it gives a slightly "soapy" taste to the fish.

Another chemical that seafood can be dipped in to preserve freshness, is citric acid. Citric acid is notorious for causing IC symptom flares. I wash seafood well before cooking to get rid of any chemicals that may linger on it. My bladder is sensitive to chemical additives, and although I've never had a problem with the small amount of citric acid on seafood, I'd rather not take chances.

Surimi

Another item of seafood to watch out for is surimi, sometimes called "imitation crab," "imitation shellfish," "kamoboko," or similar names. Surimi is chopped fish, usually Alaskan pollock, that has been made into a fine, rubbery paste and blended with other ingredients. It's those other ingredients which may cause problems for IC bladders.

Most surimi contains polyphosphate preservatives, but some also have monosodium glutamate (MSG). Although the FDA requires that surimi be labeled "imitation" in supermarkets, the law doesn't extend to restaurants. When you order "seafood salad" you may actually be getting mostly surimi.

Chinese Tuna Casserole

serves 3

Versions of this popular old recipe have been floating around for decades. My mother has been making this one since the early 70's, and it's still a family favorite.

2 c. chow mein noodles, divided ★
2 cans (6 oz.) tuna in water, drained
½ c. salted cashews
1 c. sliced celery
¼ c. chopped green onion
salt and pepper to taste
1 10-oz. can cream of mushroom soup ★
¼ c. water

Preheat oven to 375° F. Spray a 10-inch square baking dish with non-stick cooking spray or lightly coat with vegetable oil. In a bowl, combine 1 cup of the noodles, tuna, cashews, celery, onion, and salt and pepper. Combine mushroom soup and water, then pour over other ingredients. Toss lightly, then turn into baking dish. Top with remaining chow mein noodles. Bake at 375° F. for 15 minutes or until heated through.

Variations: This recipe works well with canned or leftover cooked salmon instead of tuna, and I've even made this with cubed, cooked chicken. You can also substitute cooked pasta shells or macaroni for the chow mein noodles.

Linguine with Clam Sauce

serves 3

3 cloves garlic, minced
¼ c. olive oil
3 cans (6 oz.) chopped clams ★
8 oz. clam juice (bottled) ★
2 Tbsp. dried parsley
½ tsp. basil
¼ tsp. salt
⅛ tsp. pepper
3 servings of hot, cooked linguine noodles

In medium saucepan saute the garlic in olive oil until tender. Drain chopped clams, reserving liquid from two of the cans. Add reserved liquid, clam juice, parsley, basil, salt, and pepper to the garlic. Bring to boiling, then reduce heat and simmer about 5 minutes.

Add chopped clams, heat through, and serve over linguine noodles (or your favorite hot cooked pasta).

Shrimp Variation: Omit one can of chopped clams and substitute ½ c. of tiny cooked cocktail shrimp.

> **Milder Mackerel**
>
> Some strong-tasting fish, such as mackerel, can be made milder and less "fishy" tasting by soaking the fillets in milk for a couple of hours before cooking.

San Francisco Poached Halibut

serves 2

This savory blend of oriental and maritime flavors is inspired by a dish served at San Francisco's famed restaurant, Rose Pistola.

4 medium cloves garlic, sliced
2 Tbsp. olive oil
2 fresh halibut fillets
1 8-oz. bottle clam juice ★
⅓ c. chopped fresh parsley
½ tsp. dried basil
2 oz. dry soba noodles (see note)

In a skillet, cook garlic slightly in olive oil. Pour oil and garlic into a bottom of a covered casserole dish. Use brush to spread out the oil across the bottom. Lay the fish fillets on the oil. Pour the clam juice over the fillets, then top the fillets with the chopped parsley and dried basil.

Pull the dried soba noodles from the package, separating gently, and surround the fillets with the noodles. Cover and microwave on high for 3 minutes.

Uncover and stir, pushing noodles around to make sure they are in liquid. Microwave another 3 minutes on high. Check fish. It is done if it is opaque white and flakes easily. Serve fish on a warm platter, surrounded by noodles.

Note: You can use angel hair pasta instead of soba noodles, and I've found that yellowtail or swordfish makes a wonderful alternative to halibut.

Sesame-Grilled Mahi

serves 2

2 tsp. dark oriental sesame oil
½ tsp. ground coriander
1 tsp. grated fresh ginger
2 medium cloves garlic, minced
½ lb. mahi fillets

Mix sesame oil with the coriander, ginger and garlic. Pour over the fish, cover, and chill for 3 hours. Grill over medium coals until fish flakes easily with a fork.

Salmon Bake

serves 2

This easy one-dish meal is quick to put together on those days when my bladder is flaring up.

non-stick cooking spray
3 hard-boiled eggs, chopped
1 tsp. onion salt
¼ tsp. garlic powder
½ c. chopped mushrooms
1 10-oz. can cream of mushroom soup ★
1 c. chopped celery
1 c. cooked salmon, in bite-size pieces
1½ c. chow mein noodles ★

Preheat oven to 400° F. Spray the inside of a 1½-quart covered casserole dish with non-stick cooking spray. Combine all of the ingredients in a bowl, tossing to mix well. Turn into the casserole. Cover and bake for 35 minutes. Remove cover, stir, and let stand for 5 minutes to cool slightly before serving.

Grilled Snapper with Lemon Butter

serves 3

¾ lb. red snapper fillets
2 Tbsp. butter or margarine, melted
1 tsp. grated lemon peel
pinch allspice
pinch salt

Cut snapper fillets into serving pieces if they are large. Melt butter and stir in other ingredients. Brush fish with melted butter. Grill fish about 4 or 5 inches from medium hot coals until tender and flakes easily with fork (about 20 minutes). Brush fillets with melted butter occasionally while they are grilling.

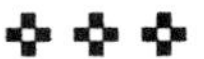

Savory Fried Fish

serves 2

2 fresh perch or sole fillets
¼ c. flour
1 tsp. garlic powder
¼ tsp. salt
dash pepper
pinch dried marjoram, crumbled

1 egg
1 Tbsp. cold water (approx.)
3 Tbsp. canola oil
2 Tbsp. olive oil

Rinse fish and pat fairly dry with towel. Mix flour, garlic powder, salt, pepper and marjoram. Beat in egg and water with fork to make a thick gravy-like consistency. Heat canola and olive oils in a skillet until a drop of water sizzles. Dip fish in batter and fry over medium heat, browning on both sides.

SOUPS AND STEWS

Busy Day Chicken-Broccoli Soup ✓

serves 2

2 c. low-sodium chicken broth ★
1 10-oz. can Campbell's Healthy Request Chicken Noodle Soup
¼ c. water
3 cloves garlic, chopped
¼ c. fresh carrots, peeled and chopped
½ c. cooked chicken
2 c. frozen broccoli florets
¼ tsp. dried thyme
salt and pepper to taste

Add the broth and canned soup to a medium saucepan with the water and bring to a simmer. Add remaining ingredients to soup, seasoning to taste with salt and pepper. Simmer for about 12 minutes before serving. Good served with crusty french bread.

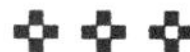

Albondigas

serves 4

This version of the traditional Mexican meatball soup is much quicker to prepare than many time-honored family recipes, but is still a hearty meal when served with warm tortillas.

1 10-oz. can condensed vegetable beef soup ★
1 10-oz. can beef broth ★
2 Tbsp. sherry (see note)
1 bay leaf
¼ tsp. dried parsley

1 lb. ground beef, lean
1 egg
¼ tsp. pepper
2 Tbsp. fresh mint, chopped fine
½ c. green onion, chopped

flour
vegetable oil, for frying
⅓ cup rice, uncooked

Empty can of vegetable soup into a blender, chopper or food processor and process for about a half a minute until the soup is almost pureed. In a medium saucepan, combine the soup, broth, sherry, bay leaf, and parsley.

Combine in a bowl the meat, egg, pepper, mint, and onion and mix well. Form meatballs about 1¼ inches across. Roll meatballs in flour to lightly coat and fry in oil until browned. As batches of meatballs are cooked, drop into the soup.

Place soup on medium heat and bring to boil. Immediately reduce heat and simmer. In hot frying pan, fry the rice in the remaining oil until lightly browned. Drop rice in the hot soup. Cover and continue simmering soup until rice is tender, about 20 minutes. Remove bay leaf and serve.

Note: The alcohol in the sherry boils off as the soup simmers but lends a distinctive flavor. Watch out for lard and bladder-provoking benzoates in tortillas if you serve them with the soup.

Cuban Bean and Vegetable Soup ✿
serves 2

2 c. cooked black beans
1 c. low-sodium chicken broth ★
1/3 c. chopped carrots
1/3 c. chopped celery
2/3 c. water
1 Tbsp. dried parsley
½ tsp. salt
½ tsp. oregano
1/8 to ¼ tsp. black pepper
1/8 tsp. garlic powder

In blender or food processor, puree one cup of the beans with a little of the chicken broth until fairly smooth, about one minute. Add whole and pureed beans, chicken broth, and remainder of ingredients to a saucepan. Bring to boil, then quickly reduce heat and simmer, covered, over low heat about 30 minutes. Serve with French bread or tortillas.

Vegetarian variation: Substitute 1 cup of vegetable broth for the chicken broth. (See Appendix B, IC Pantry, for IC-friendly brands of vegetable broth).

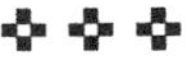

Hearty Potato Soup
serves 4

2 large russet potatoes
4 c. low-sodium chicken broth ★
1 Tbsp. sherry
2/3 c. chopped green onions
3 medium-sized cloves garlic, minced
½ c. coarsely chopped celery
½ c. finely grated carrot
3 Tbsp. butter or margarine
1 bay leaf
½ tsp. dried basil
salt to taste
1 large white rose potato

Chop russet potatoes in 1-inch chunks, add to broth with sherry and bring to a boil. Cover and simmer about 10 minutes until potatoes are soft. Meanwhile, sauté onions, garlic, celery, and carrot in butter.

Remove potatoes from broth. With a little liquid, puree in a blender or food processor. Return to simmering broth. Add sautéed vegetables, bay leaf, basil, and salt to broth.

Chop white rose potatoes in chunks about half an inch square. Stir potatoes into soup, and simmer 15 minutes more. Remove bay leaf before serving.

Note: Alcohol in sherry boils off.

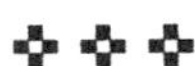

Mexican Black Bean Soup
serves 4

4 c. soaked black beans (see note)
4 c. low-sodium chicken broth ★
2 c. water
½ tsp. lemon extract

1 tsp. allspice
2 Tbsp. olive oil
10 cloves garlic, minced
½ tsp. salt
2 Tbsp. chopped chives
dash pepper, if desired
6 corn tortillas, cut in half-inch wide strips, fried in oil til crisp
sprigs of fresh cilantro, chopped

Place first 10 ingredients in a pot and bring to a boil over high heat. Reduce heat to low and let simmer, covered, for one hour.

Remove about ¾ cup of beans and a little liquid. In a blender or a food processor, puree it until fairly smooth, about 1 minute. Add it back to the soup and simmer, covered, for another half hour.

Meanwhile, fry tortilla strips in oil until crispy. Drain on paper towels. To serve, top bowls of soup with tortilla strips and about a teaspoon of chopped cilantro per bowl. Soup is also good with warmed fresh corn tortillas, or IC-Style Quesadillas (page 114).

Note: To cook black beans, you must first soak them at least 8 hours. This is a necessary step for dry, whole beans. As the bean soaks up water, a chemical reaction takes place inside it which makes it more digestible and less "gassy." (The trick works with dried split peas, too). Be sure to cover the beans with plenty of water, because they soak it up and double in volume. Use 2 cups dry beans to make 4 cups soaked beans. Throw out the soak water and rinse the beans before using.

Spring Harvest Soup

serves 3

2 Tbsp. butter
1½ c. celery, chopped fine
1 Tbsp. fresh chives (or green onion), chopped
4 c. chicken broth ★
¼ tsp. dried chervil
⅛ tsp. nutmeg
salt to taste
dash pepper, if desired
¼ c. rice

Briefly sauté celery and chives in a skillet with butter. In large saucepan combine cooked celery and chives, broth, chervil, nutmeg, salt and pepper. Bring to a boil, then add rice, cover, and reduce heat. Continue to simmer for 20 minutes.

Note: To make a more hearty soup, or for use as a one-dish meal, add half a cup of diced, cooked chicken.

Peeling a Lot of Garlic

Here's how one professional chef says he deals with the chore of peeling lots of garlic: Drop the cloves into boiling water for a few seconds to a minute and the skins will loosen and come off easily.

Autumn Vegetable Chowder ✿

serves 4

1 16-oz can yams, rinsed and drained
2½ c. low-sodium chicken broth ★
2 Tbsp. chopped fresh chives
2 Tbsp. margarine
1 c. frozen corn kernels
1½ tsp. onion salt
⅛ tsp. garlic powder
dash pepper
1 Tbsp. flour
⅓ c. low-fat milk

Puree yams in a blender or food processor with ¾ c. of the broth. Set aside.

In a soup pot, cook chives briefly in margarine, then add corn. Stir-fry a minute over medium heat. Add the yams and the remaining broth and bring to a boil. Reduce heat to low, add onion salt, garlic powder and pepper to taste. Cover and simmer for 5 minutes.

Place 1 Tbsp. of flour in a measuring cup and stir in a tablespoon of the milk to make a paste. Gradually add remaining milk. Stir into the soup and heat through.

Note: If you use a chicken broth that is not low-sodium it may be too salty, so substitute onion powder or onion flakes for the onion salt.

Vegetarian variation: Although the soup is more flavorful with chicken broth, you can use vegetable broth as a substitute. If you do, you may want to add a bit more garlic powder, chives, and pepper for added flavor.

Main dish variation: To make this versatile soup a more hearty main dish, add ⅓ c. dry rice and 1 c. diced cooked chicken when you add the yams. Then simmer for 15 minutes, covered, instead of 5 minutes. Continue the rest of the recipe as directed.

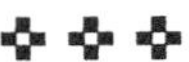

Easy Chinese Egg-Drop Soup ✓

serves 2

2 c. low-sodium chicken broth ★
2 Tbsp. carrot (or celery) finely chopped
1 tsp. onion salt
dash pepper, if desired
1 egg, beaten

Add all ingredients except egg to small saucepan and heat to boiling, then reduce heat and simmer, covered, about five minutes. Beat egg just until frothy, then pour slowly from a spoon into the hot simmering soup. Top with a bit of fresh chives if desired, and serve.

Another interesting Chinese touch is to slice a large carrot or a zucchini *very* thin, then use hors d'oeuvre cutters to make small flowers or other shapes. Float one or two on the top of the soup just before serving.

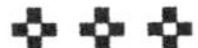

Quick Pumpkin Soup ✓

serves 4

1 medium onion, chopped
2 Tbsp. butter or margarine
1 16-oz. can low-sodium chicken broth ★
1 15-oz can cooked pumpkin
½ tsp. ground coriander
¼ tsp. salt

Sauté onion in butter until transparent. Add onion to broth in saucepan. Stir in pumpkin, coriander, and salt. Simmer 10 minutes. Garnish with chopped chives just before serving, if desired.

Easy Turkey Soup ✓

serves 1

To a can of Campbell's Healthy Request Chicken Noodle soup and ½ can of water, add ½ c. leftover cooked turkey, 1 Tbsp. chopped fresh chives, a pinch of thyme, and 2 Tbsps. finely chopped red bell pepper. Simmer 10 minutes, covered.

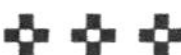

Old-Fashioned Chicken Stew

serves 2

4 chicken breasts, boned
flour
peanut oil or canola oil
4 c. water
3 c. low-sodium chicken broth ★
8 large cloves garlic, minced
2 medium onions, chopped
1 green bell pepper, chopped
½ c. carrots, sliced
8 small red new potatoes, washed and quartered
¼ tsp. pepper, optional
1 tsp. sage
1 tsp salt
2 Tbsp. dried parsley

Cut chicken into bite-sized pieces. Dredge pieces in flour and fry in oil. When slightly brown, remove and set aside. Turn off heat and add water and broth to skillet, scraping up browned bits. Pour hot liquid into a slow-cooker or electric crock pot. Add the remaining ingredients. Cook on low for 8 hours, or high for 4 hrs. (Time may vary, depending on the maker of the crock pot).

Crock-Pot Mediterranean Stew

serves 4

1 clove garlic, sliced
1 c. onion, chopped
olive oil
flour
1½ lbs. stew beef, in 1-inch cubes
1 c. zucchini or yellow squash, sliced
1 c. celery, chopped
1 c. carrots, sliced
2 c. potatoes, cubed
½ tsp. thyme
salt and pepper to taste
3 c. beef broth ★, *or* 1 tsp. beef base ★ plus 3 c. water

Saute garlic and onion in olive oil. When translucent, transfer to crockpot. Dredge chunks of beef in flour and fry in oil until browned. Add the browned beef, squash, celery, carrots, potatoes, thyme, and salt and pepper to crockpot or slow-cooker. Remove hot frying pan from stove and add beef broth, stirring and scraping up browned bits. Pour broth into crockpot, cover and cook on high for 4 hours (or until beef is cooked through and tender). Stir once while cooking.

Gulf Coast Pork Stew ✓

serves 4

1½ tsp. allspice
½ tsp. coriander
¼ tsp. ginger
¼ tsp. pepper, optional (see note)
4 pork chops, deboned

1 c. sliced onion
3 Tbsp. vegetable oil
3¼ c. chicken broth ★
1 c. red bell pepper, chopped coarsely
1 c. sliced carrot
1 c. zucchini, sliced
½ tsp. salt
2 tsp. unsulphured molasses
5 Tbsp. flour

Mix first four ingredients and rub on meat, coating completely. Seal meat in a ziplock bag or sealed container, and chill for at least 1 hour.

In a skillet, cook onion in oil until soft. Remove onion and set aside. Cut meat in bite-sized pieces and brown in oil remaining in the skillet. Remove meat and set aside.

Add chicken broth to the hot skillet, scraping up the browned bits. Pour chicken broth into a large pot, then add browned pork and cooked onions. Bring to a boil, then reduce heat, and add bell pepper and carrot. Simmer covered, over low heat for 1 hour.

Add zucchini, salt and molasses. Mix a little cold water with the flour to make a paste. Add a little of the stew liquid to the paste. Mix and return to stew pot. Cover and simmer half an hour more. Serve over noodles or in bowls with warm french bread.

Note: For those on a low-oxalate diet, the pepper can be reduced or omitted.

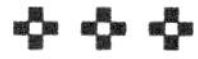

A New Mouse in the Kitchen

A new kitchen tool can help IC cooks collect and store their recipes, find them instantly, and even analyze them for nutritional content. This 6-inch high kitchen computer allows you to type in foods you have on hand, and then it finds recipes that use those items. Unlike bulky computers, it takes up only a tiny piece of counter space and the screen is tilted back at an angle for comfortable reading. Called *Kitchen Assistant*, it's featured in several catalogs, including Spiegel.

Beef Stew with Allspice
serves 3

1½ lbs. stew beef, in 1-inch cubes
½ c. flour
vegetable oil
2¾ c. water
2 Tbsp. sherry

2 cloves garlic, minced
2 bay leaves
1 tsp. salt
½ tsp. sugar
¼ tsp. pepper
¼ tsp. allspice
¼ c. celery chopped fine
½ c. sliced carrots
1½ c. red potatoes, in 1-inch cubes
1 Tbsp. fresh chives, chopped

Dredge beef in flour and fry in oil until browned. Add water to frying pan, scraping up browned bits. Pour into a large pot, add beef and sherry, then bring to a boil. Reduce heat to simmer and add garlic, bay leaves, salt, sugar, pepper and allspice. Simmer covered for 1½ hours. Add last four ingredients and simmer covered, another ½ hour. Remove bay leaves and serve.

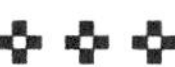

Pollo de Santa Cruz ✓
serves 4

3 chicken half-breasts, deboned
flour
olive oil
2 c. low-sodium chicken broth ★
1 c. water
2 c. boiling potatoes, in 1-inch chunks

6 cloves garlic, sliced
1¼ tsp. onion salt
1½ tsp. dried parsley or chervil
½ tsp. dried oregano
¼ tsp. dried thyme

1 c. pitted black olives
1 8-oz. can artichoke hearts, drained and rinsed (see note)

¼ tsp. orange extract

Chop chicken in bite-sized pieces and dredge in flour. In a skillet, brown chicken pieces in olive oil. Remove chicken. Add broth to hot skillet, scraping up browned bits. Pour the broth in a large soup pot and add chicken, potatoes, garlic, onion salt and spices. Cover and simmer 1 hour. Add olives, artichoke hearts, and extract. Simmer another ½ hour.

Note: Be sure to drain and rinse the artichoke hearts well. Citric acid may have been added to the water in the can.

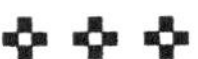

Hearty Beef Stew ✓

serves 3

This filling beef stew is perfect for those flare days when you don't want to risk provoking an already irritated bladder. Relatively bland, and featuring only the most innocuous ingredients, it is still a tasty and protein-packed meal.

1 lb. stew beef, cubed
flour
3 Tbsp. olive oil
4 c. water
½ tsp. garlic powder
¼ tsp. salt
1 tsp. dried chervil
2 bay leaves
1 c. sliced carrots
6 new red potatoes, cut in chunks
dash pepper, (see note)

Dredge beef chunks in flour and shake off excess. In a skillet, brown beef in olive oil. Remove beef and place in a 2-quart covered saucepan.

Pour water into the hot skillet and scrape up the browned bits with a spatula. Pour into the saucepan with the meat. Add garlic powder, salt, chervil, bay leaves, carrots and potatoes to the meat.

Bring to a boil, then cover, reduce to a simmer and cook 1 hour. Stir in a little flour and water to thicken if needed, removing bay leaves before serving. (This is good served with biscuits or broiled muenster cheese-topped french bread).

Note: To add more zip (on days when your bladder feels better), stir in a dash of pepper, ¼ cup chopped green onion or chives, and ¼cup chopped celery (only if you're not on a low-oxalate diet) with the carrots and potatoes.

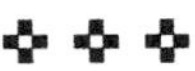

VEGETABLES, SALADS AND SIDE DISHES

Asparagus Russe ✿
serves 3

1 lb. fresh asparagus
½ c. bread crumbs, unseasoned
1 hard-cooked egg, chopped
¼ c. margarine or butter
2 Tbsp. chopped fresh parsley

Clean and trim asparagus, then steam or boil until tender. Drain and keep warm. Spread bread crumbs on tray in toaster oven or on cookie sheet in conventional oven. Toast at 400° F. until brown. (Watch carefully to avoid scorching). Heat butter in a small pan, add bread crumbs, chopped egg, parsley. Spoon over asparagus and serve.

Quick Asparagus Toppers ✿✓

Butter sauce

Pour melted butter over hot, cooked asparagus and top with finely chopped almonds.

Mushroom sauce

Sauté fresh, sliced mushrooms in butter, add a dash of garlic powder and spoon over hot, cooked asparagus.

Cheese melt

Melt shredded muenster cheese over cooked asparagus.

Nutmeg Green Beans ✿
serves 2

1½ c. frozen, julienne-cut green beans
1 Tbsp. butter
⅛ tsp. ground nutmeg

Steam green beans until tender, then drain thoroughly. In a small saucepan melt butter over low heat, add nutmeg and stir a few seconds to distribute the flavor. Add green beans, stirring to coat, and cover. Cook for an additional minute or two to let beans heat through.

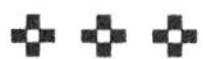

Green Beans with Coriander ✿
serves 4

2 c. fresh green beans, sliced
2 medium cloves garlic, minced
2 Tbsp. olive oil
½ tsp. coriander, ground

Cook green beans in water until tender. Drain well and set aside, keeping warm. In saucepan, over medium heat, sauté minced garlic for about 30 seconds in the olive oil, just until tender. Add the green beans and coriander, tossing to coat and warm through.

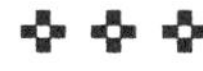

Greener Green Beans

With the exception of the Southwest, where the water is often hard and alkaline, most places have slightly acid tap water. If your water is very acid, you may see your green beans turn an unappetizing gray when they are cooked.

Because green beans are a relatively "safe" food for most IC patients to eat, we don't think of them as having acids. They do contain some natural acids though, and those food acids react with the beans' chlorophyll when they are cooked in hot water. This reaction makes the beans turn gray. Slightly acid cooking water can accelerate the graying process.

To help keep that vibrant green color, you can cook them without a lid, since the lid traps and concentrates the acids which might otherwise evaporate with the water. There is a downside to cooking without a lid, though: loss of vitamin content. You will have to cook the beans longer, and the longer you cook vegetables, the more vitamins are lost.

Another strategy to keep beans green, is to add a little baking soda to the water. Just a tiny pinch should do the trick. But be careful, too much baking soda will make the beans soft and mushy.

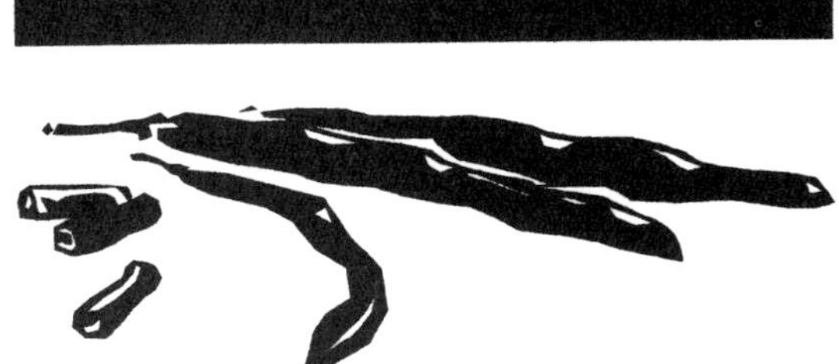

Rosemary Green Beans ✿

serves 2

½ lb. fresh green beans
2 tsp. margarine
3 Tbsp. onion, chopped
⅛ tsp. garlic powder
1 dash salt
¼ tsp. dried rosemary, crushed
⅛ tsp. dried basil, crushed

Wash green beans and trim off ends. Cook whole beans until tender (about 20 minutes). Drain well. In skillet or large saucepan over low heat, melt margarine and sauté onions until clear. Quickly stir in garlic powder, salt and herbs, then add beans. Toss gently to coat. Cover and heat through before serving.

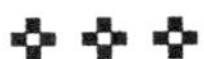

Green Beans with Pecans ✿

serves 2

For those able to eat a few pecans, this variation on the almond-green bean combination is just too delicious to pass up!

1 c. frozen green beans, julliene-sliced
½ Tbsp. butter or margarine
1 Tbsp. fresh parsley, chopped
2 Tbsp. fresh chives, snipped
2 Tbsp. pecans, finely chopped
dash salt and pepper (optional)

Cook green beans until tender, drain well. In saucepan, melt butter and add parsley, chives and pecans. Stir for one minute over low heat, just to cook the chives. Add beans to the pecans and heat through while stirring, about another minute or so. Add dash of salt and pepper if desired, and serve.

Cashew variation: If you can't eat pecans, try substituting cashews.

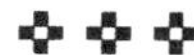

Golden Fried Eggplant ✿

serves 4

1 medium eggplant
1 egg, beaten
½ c. unseasoned dry bread crumbs
1 Tbsp. marjoram
½ tsp. garlic powder
¼ tsp. salt
flour
cooking oil (see note)

Peel, then slice eggplant crosswise into very thin (⅛-inch) rounds. Beat egg in a small bowl. In another bowl, combine crumbs with marjoram, garlic powder, and salt, mixing well. Coat eggplant with flour, shaking off excess, then dip in egg. Roll in bread crumbs. Heat oil in a skillet over medium heat, and fry eggplant until golden brown, turning once. Drain on paper towels and serve.

Note: Olive oil adds to the flavor, but it scorches easily.

Carolina Tarragon Carrots ✿✓

serves 2

2 c. sliced, peeled carrots
⅛ tsp. salt
2 Tbsp. butter or margarine
½ tsp. dried tarragon

Steam or boil sliced carrots until tender and drain well. Set aside and keep warm.

In medium saucepan, melt butter and add salt. Add dried tarragon to the buttter and stir well. Cook over low heat for about a minute, being careful not to burn the butter. Add drained carrots and toss gently to coat.

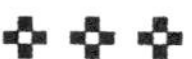

Minted Baby Carrots ✿✓

serves 4

2 c. baby carrots, washed and pared
dash salt
water
1 Tbsp. butter or margarine
1 Tbsp. sugar
1 Tbsp. fresh mint leaves, chopped

Place carrots in skillet and add water and salt to a depth of about half an inch. Cover and simmer until tender, about 10 minutes. When done, pour off any leftover water and add butter to skillet with carrots. Sauté over low heat until butter is melted. Add the sugar and mint. Continue cooking until the carrots are glazed, turning and stirring frequently.

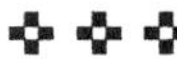

Golden Carrot Fritters ✿✓

serves 2

1 c. grated carrot, pressed (about 4 large carrots)

1 egg

dash salt

¼ tsp. coriander

3 Tbsp. flour

cooking oil or margarine

Optional carrot-honey sauce:

2 Tbsp. butter

⅛ tsp. ground ginger

1 tsp. honey

2 tsp. cornstarch

reserved carrot juice

Grate carrots coarsely, then press through a strainer to remove most of the juice. Reserve juice, measure grated carrot. Beat egg slightly and add carrot, salt, coriander and flour.

In skillet, heat oil. Spoon carrot mixture in two portions in skillet, patting with back of spatula to flatten into pancake shape. Place lid on skillet and fry over medium heat about 2 minutes. Turn fritters and fry uncovered another minute or so until batter is set and fritter is golden. Serve without sauce, or keep warm while making sauce.

For sauce: In small saucepan melt butter and add ginger, honey and cornstarch. Stir until thoroughly mixed. Add water to carrot juice to make ¼ cup.

Add juice to butter mixture, return to heat, stirring until thick. When carrot juice is thickened, pour over fritters and serve.

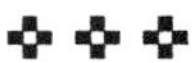

Corn with Two Rices 

serves 3

¼ c. wild rice

¼ c. long-grain white rice

1 Tbsp. margarine

1½ c. water

1 Tbsp. olive oil

2 cloves garlic, minced

2 c. frozen corn kernels

1 Tbsp. dried basil

salt and pepper to taste

In covered saucepan, cook wild rice, white rice, and margarine in water until water is absorbed and rice is done (about half an hour). In a skillet, saute minced garlic in the olive oil for a few seconds, just til tender.

Add frozen corn and cooked rices to the skillet, stirring to coat. Sprinkle basil on top and add about 2 Tbsp. of water. Cover and simmer over medium to low heat for 5 to 6 minutes. Stir to fluff rice and serve.

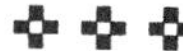

Less Cauliflower and Cabbage Aroma

If you enjoy cooked cabbage but despise the unpleasant odor that it leaves in your house, here are a couple of strategies that may help. First, try cooking cabbage as little time as possible. Steaming or lightly cooking in oil or butter is preferable to long periods of boiling. As cabbage cooks it emits hydrogen sulfide, a gas which is also produced by rotten eggs. The amount of gas which is being produced by the cabbage increases as it cooks longer. Cauliflower has much the same odor problem. Traditionally, chefs have handled it this way: Tear a piece of fresh french bread in pieces and let the chunks float on the surface of the water that the cauliflower or cabbage is cooking in (or if steaming, let the whole piece sit on top of the cabbage). Remove carefully before serving. The bread will absorb some of the offensive odor.

Spiced Creamed Corn 

serves 3

1 16-oz. can low-salt, cream-style corn ★
1/8 tsp. ground allspice
dash salt

Heat all ingredients in a small saucepan over low to medium heat, stirring occasionally to avoid scorching. Serve when hot and bubbly.

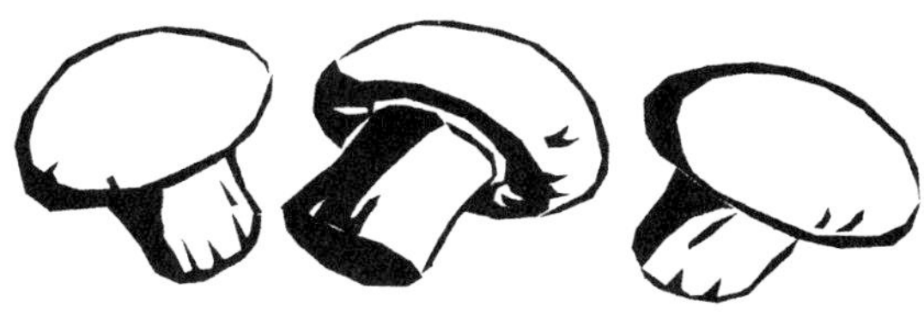

Mushrooms with Garlic ✿✓

serves 2

3 Tbsp. olive oil
4 cloves garlic, medium sized
2 c. sliced mushrooms
dash salt

Heat oil in skillet, slice garlic thinly. Saute garlic slices a few seconds, stirring to coat, then add mushroom slices and salt. Stir to coat mushrooms and cover.

Continue cooking, stirring occasionally, over low to medium heat about 5 minutes until mushrooms are cooked through. (It is especially good served over steaks).

Sweet-Tooth Baked Squash ✿

serves 2

1 small acorn squash
¼ c. butter or margarine, melted
⅛ tsp. mace
3 Tbsp. brown sugar, firmly packed
3 Tbsp. nuts, chopped fine (optional)

Carefully wash acorn squash, remove seeds, and cut in rings about one inch thick. Coat the bottom of a shallow baking dish with a little butter and place squash rings in the dish, slightly overlapping.

Pour remaining melted butter over squash rings. Sprinkle evenly with mace and brown sugar. Top with nuts, if desired. Cover and bake at 350° F. until squash is tender, about 35 minutes.

Note: Walnuts or pecans are best in this recipe, but if you can't tolerate them, cashews are a delicious crunchy addition.

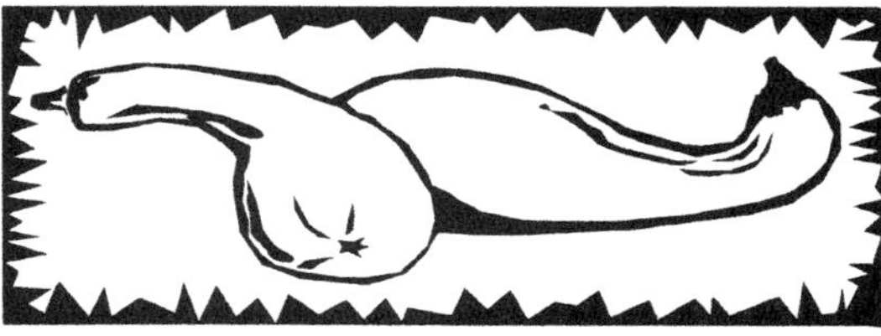

Dilled Zucchini Squash ✿✓

serves 2

1 Tbsp. butter or margarine
2 c. zucchini, sliced
2 Tbsp. parsley, dried
1 pinch dill weed, dried
salt to taste

In skillet over low to medium heat, melt butter and add zucchini. Cover and cook for 5 minutes stirring occasionally. Add parsley, dill, and salt. Stir and cook about 5 more minutes until squash is tender. Serve immediately.

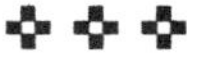

Summer Squash and Mushrooms ✿

serves 4

12 to 14 fresh mushrooms
4 yellow crookneck squash, sliced
3 Tbsp. butter or margarine
2 Tbsp. olive oil
4 large cloves garlic, minced
1 tsp. chopped chives
salt, to taste

Chop mushrooms in half-inch cubes. Slice squash in circles, about a quarter of an inch thick. Melt butter with olive oil in skillet over medium heat.

Add squash, minced garlic and mushrooms, stirring to coat. Cover and cook til tender, about 3 minutes. Add chives and sauté, stirring for another minute, just to heat. Season to taste and serve.

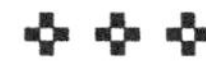

Patty Pan Squash with Almonds ✿

serves 4

2 Tbsp. almonds, ground fine
4 large patty pan squash
5 Tbsp. margarine
½ tsp. salt
dash pepper
3 cloves garlic, minced
½ tsp. basil

Grind or chop almonds finely, trim ends and cut squash in ¼-inch thick chunks. Melt margarine in skillet over medium to low heat, add salt and pepper. Add squash to skillet, cover and stir occasionally for about 5 minutes. When squash is tender, add garlic, basil and almonds. Cook about a minute more. Remove with slotted spoon to serving bowl.

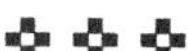

Zucchini Santa Fe ✿✓

serves 3

1 large red bell pepper
3 medium zucchini
2 Tbsp. butter
½ tsp. poppy seeds
¼ tsp. onion salt

Slice pepper in strips. Wash zucchini, cut off stem and flower ends. Cut zucchini in long thin strips, or thin circles. Heat butter in skillet, add zucchini, and bell pepper. Cover and cook on low to medium heat for about 5 minutes.

Add poppy seed and onion salt, stir vegetables and continue cooking until vegetables are soft and moisture in pan is absorbed.

Getting the Most From Vegetables

Healthy servings of vegetables can increase your daily intake of fiber and vitamins and doctors are recommending that Americans include more in their diet. Here are some ideas to increase the nutritional value of cooked vegetables:

- Use a minimum amount of water. Cook vegetables just to the "tender-crisp" stage so they look and taste the best. This will also help retain the vitamins.
- Scrub new red potatoes, cook, and serve unpeeled for more fiber.
- Try cooking starchy vegetables like potatoes or turnips in broth instead of water. It will add to the flavor and also the nutrient value of the vegetable.
- If you like greens (turnip, mustard, kale, or collards) cooked with bacon or ham, here is a lower-fat and more IC-safe method to try: Make meat broth ahead of time and refrigerate. The fat will be a solid on top and can be easily removed. You can freeze the broth (or refrigerate one or two days) and use it later for cooking greens.

Sun-Dried Tomatoes

Sun-dried plum tomatoes are allowed to ripen before drying, thus converting a substantial amount of their acidity to fruit sugars. They are then packed in oil, usually without adding citric acid or artificial preservatives. Some IC patients who cannot tolerate eating cooked tomatoes, tomato sauces or even raw low-acid tomatoes, can eat small amounts of sun-dried tomatoes. They are a tasty and excellent way to give some color to your favorite dishes. Try some on salads, or on top of cooked vegetables!

Molded Melon Salad ✿

serves 4

1½ c. honeydew melon (or half crenshaw and half honeydew) in one-inch chunks
2 envelopes unflavored gelatin
¼ c. cold water
1¼ c. sugar
2½ c. water
⅓ c. chopped mint, loosely packed
⅛ tsp. turmeric
2½ tsp. finely grated orange peel
¼ tsp. lemon extract
dash salt

Cut melon and place in refirgerator to chill while making salad. Soften the gelatin in the ¼ c. cold water (about 5 minutes).

In a small saucepan, bring the sugar and 2½ cups water to a boil, then remove from heat immediately. Add softened gelatin to the sugar water, stirring until blended. Stir in mint and turmeric and set aside to cool. When cooled (about 15 minutes), strain the mixture and remove and discard mint.

Add orange peel, lemon extract, salt. Chill in refrigerator until slightly thickened (about 10 minutes, check often because it sets up quickly).

Fold in melon chunks, scoop into individual molds or a one-quart mold. Chill until firm. Unmold on crisp lettuce to serve.

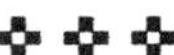

Melon-Blueberry Fruit Salad ✿

serves 4

3½ c. honeydew melon, cut in chunks
1 c. ripe, fresh blueberries
¼ tsp. lemon extract

4 tsp. honey
¼ tsp. ground coriander
¼ tsp. ground nutmeg

Cut melon into chunks and place in bowl with blueberries. Add extract, honey and spices, mix well with a large spoon. Chill before serving.

Watermelon Kebobs with Honey-Basil Sauce ✿✓

serves 4

This is a fun dish to serve at barbecues alongside the usual beef-and-vegetable kebobs... and if you can't eat watermelon, try it with honeydew!

2 Tbsp. water
1½ tsp. cornstarch
3 Tbsp.honey
3 Tbsp. cooking sherry
¼ c. finely chopped fresh basil
4 bamboo skewers
seedless watermelon, chilled

Combine water and cornstarch in a small saucepan, stirring to mix thoroughly. Add honey and sherry. Bring to boiling to evaporate alcohol. Boil for one minute while stirring. Remove from heat and add basil. Chill. Meanwhile, cut watermelon in chunks, thread on bamboo skewers, and place kebobs on a plate. Just before serving, drain juice from kebobs and dry with paper towels. Arrange on a platter, drizzle cold basil sauce over kebobs and serve.

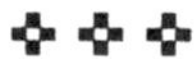

Carrot Salad with Honey Dressing ✿

serves 4

2 c. grated carrot
2 tsp. fresh mint, finely chopped
4 tsp. dried parsley
2 Tbsp. raisins (optional)
2 tsp. canola oil
½ tsp. ground coriander
2 tsp. honey
dash salt

Mix grated carrot, mint, parsley, and raisins if desired, in a salad bowl.

Combine oil, coriander, honey, and salt, whisking together until blended. Pour over salad, tossing to blend. Chill and serve.

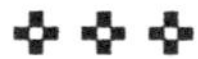

Cucumber and Dill Salad ✿

serves 3

1 large cucumber
salt
⅓ c. "Sour Cream" Base (see recipe, page 187)
2 Tbsp. chopped chives
1 Tbsp. finely chopped red bell pepper
½ tsp. dried dillweed
½ tsp. onion salt

⅛ tsp. black pepper

Peel and slice cucumber in thin slices. Arrange cucumber on a paper towel. Sprinkle with the salt, cover with another towel, and let them sit for 30 to 35 minutes. Dry off the cucumber. Combine the "sour cream" base, chives, bell pepper, dillweed, onion salt and pepper in a bowl. Pour over cucumbers, toss, and refrigerate about 30 minutes before serving.

Note: If your bladder can tolerate a very small amount of vinegar, try adding ¼ tsp., a few drops at a time, to enhance the flavor. (Green onions make the dish zestier too, if you can tolerate a little).

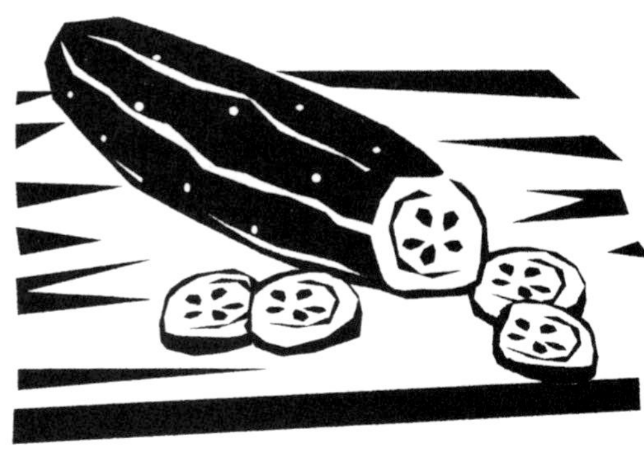

Low-Fat Ranch Dressing ✿

serves 3

- ⅔ c. "Sour Cream" Base (see recipe in Miscellaneous section)
- 1 tsp. garlic powder
- ½ tsp. salt
- ¼ tsp. pepper
- 1 tsp. basil
- 1 tsp. olive oil
- ¼ to ½ c. low-fat milk

Place all the ingredients except the milk in a bowl. Whisk in ¼ c. of the milk. Keep adding milk until it becomes the right consistency, while stirring.

Chill for an hour before serving to let flavors blend.

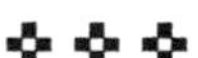

Mykonos Salad 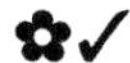

serves 4

- 1 large bell pepper (see variation)
- 5 radishes
- 1 cucumber
- 3 c. shredded romaine lettuce
- ⅓ c. sliced black olives, rinsed and drained
- ¼ c. crumbled feta cheese (see note)
- 2 Tbsp. olive oil
- ¾ tsp. dried oregano
- ½ tsp. onion salt
- ⅛ tsp. black pepper (see variation)

Slice radishes and chop bell pepper coarsely. Peel cucumber, then cut in half lengthwise and scoop out the seeds. Slice into thin crescents.

Combine lettuce, cucumber, radish, olives, and cheese in a large salad bowl, tossing gently to mix. In a small cup, combine olive oil, oregano, onion salt, and pepper. Just before serving stir oil and spices, then pour over the salad tossing to coat.

Note: Feta cheese is an unripened Greek cheese that is "pickled" in salt. (See the section on cheese in Part 1, A

Closer Look at Some Problem Foods). Chunks of Farmer cheese or mozzarella work well in this salad also.

Low-oxalate variation: Use a red, not green, bell pepper and cut amount of it by half. Omit black pepper.

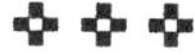

Naked Pizza Salad 

serves 4 or 5

This salad takes its name from the zesty pizza ingredients— crusty bread, Italian cheese, and sun-dried tomatoes— which lurk among the leafy greens. The generous amounts of cheese and croutons give each bite a lively flavor even when served "naked"— without dressing.

¼ head boston lettuce

½ head red leaf lettuce

8 radishes. sliced

1 bell pepper, thinly sliced (see note)

⅓ c. Marinated Mozzarella Bits (see recipe that follows)

2 small sun-dried tomatoes in oil, drained and chopped (optional, see note)

⅓ c. Italian Salad Croutons (see recipe that follows)

Tear letttuce into bite-sized pieces and combine with other ingredients in a salad bowl, adding croutons just before serving.

Note: Some IC patients can eat oil-packed sun-dried tomatoes, even though fresh tomatoes or tomato sauce causes them discomfort. To avoid high-oxalate foods, use a red bell pepper, instead of a green one, or substitute cucumber.

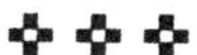

Marinated Mozzarella Bits ✿✓

2 oz. low-fat Mozzarella cheese

2 cloves garlic, pressed

¼ c. olive oil

3 Tbsp. chopped fresh basil

2 Tbsp. dried parsley or chervil (see note)

If your cheese is in a block, cut cheese into half-inch cubes. If it's pre-sliced in thin slices, just use the slices, whole. Combine all in a ziplock bag and refrigerate 8 to 24 hours.

When done marinating, wipe the excess oil and spices off the cheese slices. You can use hors d'oeuvre cutters to cut fancy shapes from sliced cheese, or just cut in squares. Store in closed container in refrigerator until ready to use.

Note: If you're avoiding high-oxalate foods, you have two options: leave out the parsley, and increase the basil by 1 tablespoon, *or* try chervil instead of the parsley.

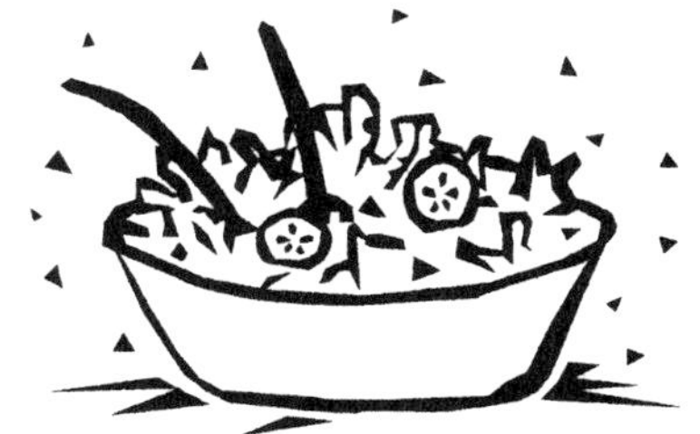

Italian Salad Croutons ✿✓

makes 2 cups croutons

2 c. stale bread cubes (see note)
2 Tbsp. olive oil
1 clove pressed garlic
dash salt and pepper, if desired
⅛ tsp. ground oregano

Cut french bread or whole wheat bread into ¾-inch cubes. Combine remaining ingredients in a bowl. Tip bowl to coat the bowl with the oil. Add bread and toss. Oil a rimmed cookie sheet, then spread out bread on sheet. Bake at 375° F. for about 6 to 12 minutes, stirring every 3 minutes or so. Watch carefully, because these burn easily. (They can be stored dry and refrigerated for up to 10 days).

Note: To make fresh bread "stale," put slices in oven or toaster just until slightly dried out. Two slices of store-bought bread make about a cup of cubes.

Salad Strategies

After many years of struggling to find a salad compromise, I have to admit that nothing will replace the taste of a favorite salad dressing. But on the other hand, salads don't have to be boring and tasteless either. There are several ways to perk up IC-safe salads.

First, evaluate the sensitivity of your bladder. Can you have a small amount of vinegar? Or none at all? Making your own dressings from scratch will allow you to experiment with reducing the amount of acid. Your homemade dressing can have less vinegar than store-bought products. For some people, just reducing the acid level is sufficient. Of the readily available commercial products, I find that I can sometimes have *Newman's Own Olive Oil and Vinegar* dressing. It seems to have less vinegar than some others, and has no MSG.

If you find you can't tolerate any acid at all, don't despair. There are other ways you can give your salads a little zing:

Distraction works wonders

Make the salad more flavorful in terms of what you put in it. Radishes or a little bit of chopped chives can perk it up. Ditto for unripened cheeses, croutons, black olives, sunflower seeds, some brands of imitation bacon bits (see Appendix B), broken snack crackers, bits of fresh basil leaf, grilled fish or chicken, sun-dried tomatoes, etc, etc. Pick interesting textures and zesty flavors that will distract your taste buds from the less glamorous greens. Pick stronger tasting vegetables such as broccoli or turnips to pair with less tasty ones. (Beware of vegetables in the cabbage family if you also have IBS. The gas they cause may trigger intestinal symptoms unless you also use a product such as Beano). Throw in bits of red cabbage or radicchio to add visual interest. Experiment with odd-colored bell peppers.

Get weird

Try to imagine that you're from Mars and never saw a salad before. You don't know the "rules" of what you can put in it. Then think of what might taste good with the greens. Remember making all kinds of "concoctions" of food when you were a kid? Kids are great idea generators. Can you tolerate peanut butter?...it tastes good on stuffed celery sticks, so why not on a chopped celery and lettuce salad????

Got a barbecue sauce your bladder can tolerate? Give it a try on lettuce and bell pepper...Not bad! Try crazy combinations... you have nothing to lose!

The "OPEC" alternative— just oil

Plain oil on lettuce is slippery, not flavorful, and for those watching their weight or cholesterol, too much oil means trouble. But as an occasional and sparingly-used alternative, flavored oils can lend a subtle enhancement to salad greens. Walnut oil and olive oil are tasty by themselves. Try oils flavored with herbs or vegetables. (There are ready-made herb-flavored oils on the market, but many brands have chile peppers or something "hot" in them. It may be best to make them yourself).

Garlic flavored oil is easy to make, and will keep for at least three weeks in the refrigerator. (Oils with herbs may turn a bit cloudy at the low refrigerator temperatures, but will taste fine.) Be sure not to drown the salad in flavored oil because oil *is* heavy. Just a *very* light drizzle does the trick.

Use herbs creatively

Another alternative is to forego both the acid and the oil of salad dressings, and just use the herbs. Dry crumbled oregano, marjoram, basil, or dill sprinkled on a moist salad and tossed, brings the greens to life. Chopped fresh basil, cilantro, parsley, or other herbs can enliven the taste too. Fresh nasturium flowers add a bit of color and a peppery taste, while chive flowers add an onion-y flavor without onions.

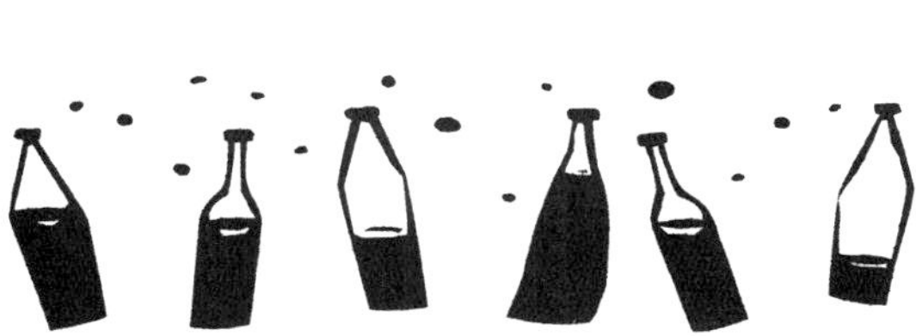

Basil-Flavored Olive Oil 

You'll find this oil in the gourmet section of your market, priced accordingly, or you can easily make it yourself for much less money. I love to fry hash browns or omelets in this. Try tossing a salad of lettuce, alfalfa sprouts, and feta cheese with a tiny splash of this.

1 c. extra virgin olive oil
1 medium clove garlic, peeled
½ c. fresh basil leaves. loosely packed

Pour the oil in a small saucepan and add whole garlic cloves and basil. Cook over low to medium heat until the cloves of garlic turn a light golden brown. Set the pan of oil aside to cool. When room temperature, pour the mixture into a clean container, making sure the lid is airtight. Store in the refrigerator. After 3 days, strain out the garlic and basil, and it is ready to use. You can keep it refrigerated for about 3 weeks.

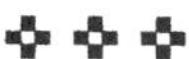

Roasted Garlic Oil 

I cook mushrooms and fry potatoes in this delicious oil, as well as add a light drizzle to tossed salads.

1 c. light olive oil or canola oil
6 medium cloves garlic, peeled

Place the oil in a small saucepan and add whole garlic cloves. Cook over low to medium heat until the cloves of garlic turn a light golden brown. Set the pan of oil aside to cool. When it is at room temperature, pour into a clean container, making sure the lid is airtight. Store in the refrigerator. You can keep it refrigerated for 3 or 4 weeks.

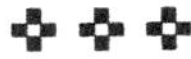

Malaysian Ginger Oil ✿

Here is another flavorful and versatile oil. It adds a subtle oriental flavor to salads with bean sprouts, or to fried rice. I have also mixed it with a little of the low-sodium soy sauce I can tolerate, and used that as a light sauce for steamed snow peas. Be sure to use Asian sesame oil, which is a dark molasses-brown color. You will proabably find it in in the ethnic foods section of the supermarket, or in one of the specialty markets listed in the back of the book.

3 Tbsp. Asian sesame oil
1¼ c. canola oil
5 medium garlic cloves, peeled
4 green peppercorns (optional)
1 piece of fresh ginger, peeled (about 2 inches long)
2 drops lemon extract

Pour the oil in a small saucepan and place over medium heat. Add the remaining ingredients. Cover and cook, stirring and checking every so often, until garlic turns a golden brown. Set aside, uncovered, to let cool to room temperature.

When cooled, remove just the garlic cloves and pour everything else into a very clean container with an airtight lid. (The less air trapped, the better, since oxygen makes oil become rancid). Store in the refrigerator and, after one week, remove the ginger and peppercorns. The oil is then ready to use and can be kept refrigerated for three or four weeks.

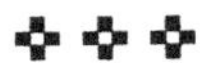

Potate Roma ✓

serves 4

1¼ lbs. (2 or 3 medium-sized) russet potatoes
2 c. chicken broth ★
½ c. water
2 cloves garlic, peeled
¼ c. 2% lowfat milk, warmed
2 Tbsp. butter
⅛ tsp. dried basil
salt to taste
pepper (optional)

Peel and quarter the potatoes. In a large saucepan combine potatoes, broth, water and garlic. Bring to a boil, then reduce heat, cover, and simmer until potatoes are very soft when pierced with a fork, about 30 minutes. Drain garlic and potatoes, reserving ¼ cup broth. Mash potatoes with butter, basil, milk, and ¼ cup of reserved broth. (The amount of broth is approximate. Add more broth for creamier potatoes). Season with salt and pepper.

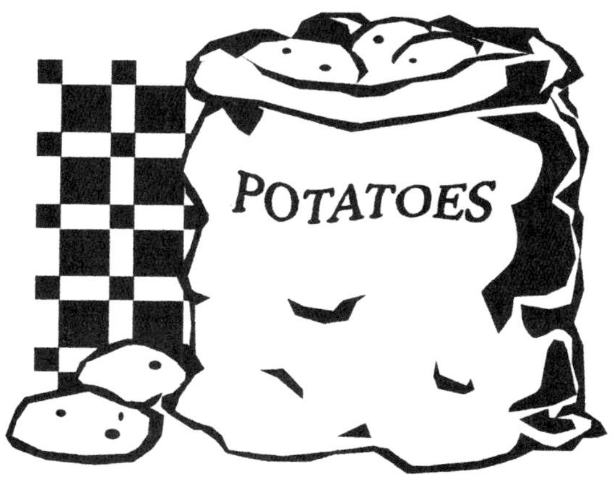

Rosemary Roasted Potatoes ✿✓

serves 4

4 to 6 new red potatoes
3 Tbsp. olive oil
1 garlic clove, minced
¼ tsp. salt
1 Tbsp. chives, fresh chopped
1 tsp. dried rosemary, slightly crushed
dash pepper (see note)

Preheat oven to 400° F. and scrub potatoes. Cut in quarters (for large) or halves (for smaller ones). Add olive oil to a cast-iron skillet and heat.

When hot, add garlic, potatoes and salt, stirring to coat thoroughly. Place skillet in oven and bake at 400° F. until potatoes are slightly soft, about 20 min.

Remove from oven and add chives, rosemary and pepper, stirring to coat. Return to oven for about 10 or 15 minutes more until potatoes are soft.

Note: For a low-oxalate version, omit the pepper. If you don't have a cast-iron skillet, use a regular skillet to brown the potatoes, then transfer the hot oil and potatoes to a rimmed cookie sheet or a metal baking pan.

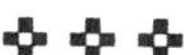

Skillet Roasted Potatoes ✿✓

serves 4

¼ c. olive oil
3 large white boiling potatoes, pared
½ tsp. salt

1 Tbsp. chopped onion
pinch dried parsley
½ teaspon dried thyme
2 Tbsp. green bell pepper, finely chopped

Preheat oven to 400° F. Cut the potatoes in chunks, about an inch across. Add olive oil to a cast-iron skillet and heat until a drop of water sizzles, but don't let oil smoke. When skillet is hot, add potatoes and salt, stirring to coat thoroughly. Using an oven mitt, place skillet in oven. Let bake at 400° F. until potatoes are slightly soft, about 15-20 minutes.

Carefully remove from oven and quickly add onion, parsley, thyme, and bell pepper, stirring to coat. Return to oven for 10 minutes more until potatoes are soft and lightly browned.

Low-oxalate variation: Substitute dried chervil for the dried parsley, and chopped red bell pepper for the green bell pepper (or omit bell pepper).

Angel Hair with Squash ✿

serves 4

6 medium crookneck squash or 4 large patty pan squash
8 Tbsp. butter or margarine
¼ tsp. pepper
¼ tsp. salt
1 tsp. fresh lemon peel, grated
angel hair pasta, cooked and kept warm

Slice squash thinly. In skillet melt butter and add squash, pepper and salt. Cook, stirring occasionally to prevent sticking. When squash is tender, add grated lemon peel, tossing gently to coat.

Spoon squash and sauce over angel hair pasta and serve.

Low-oxalate variation: Omit the pepper and lemon peel. Use zucchini instead of yellow squash or patty pan squash. Add ¼ tsp. of lemon extract and toss, just before serving.

Southern-Style Dirty Rice

serves 4

⅔ c. onion, chopped
½ c. finely diced bell pepper
¼ c. chopped celery
1 Tbsp. cooking oil or margarine
salt and pepper to taste
⅔ c. long-grain white rice
1⅔ c. chicken broth ★

In a skillet, cook the onion, bell pepper and celery in the oil until soft. Stir in salt and pepper, and the rice. Stir to coat rice. Add broth and bring to a boil. Reduce heat and simmer, covered, about 30 minutes until all the liquid has been absorbed.

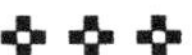

Classic Wild Rice Pilaf ✓

serves 4

¾ c. wild rice
⅓ c. finely chopped green onion
1 8-oz. can mushrooms, drained
2 Tbsp. butter or margarine
¼ c. white rice
4 c. beef broth ★
2 Tbsp. chopped fresh parsley (see note)
pinch garlic powder
salt and pepper to tatse

Rinse wild rice in cold water. Drain. In a saucepan, cook onion and mushrooms in butter until soft. Add the two rices and stir to coat with melted butter. Add the broth, parsley, garlic powder, and salt and pepper if desired. Bring to a boil, then simmer uncovered about 50 minutes, until moisture is absorbed (cover if the moisture is evaporating too fast). Fluff the rice with a fork and turn into a serving bowl.

Note: For a low-oxalate version, omit parsley and add 1 Tbsp. dried chervil last five minutes of cooking.

Secret of Perfect Pilafs

Technique makes the difference between a fluffy pilaf and a sticky mess. Suzanne, who worked in North Africa and whose husband is from the Middle East, makes pilafs for her family regularly. She put me on to this trick: first toss the uncooked rice, couscous, or other grain with a little melted butter or oil. Use just enough to lightly coat the grains. Then when you cook the grains with liquid, they soften, but don't stick together in a gluey mass.

Quick Broccoli Couscous 

serves 2

olive oil
1 bell pepper, seeded, and sliced in strips
1 c. dry couscous
2 c. chicken broth ★
¼ tsp. dried oregano
4 c. frozen broccoli flowerets
2 Tbsp. chopped almonds

Add a tespoon or so of olive oil to a saucepan and cook bell pepper strips until limp. Turn heat off under the pan, remove the bell pepper and reserve. Add dry couscous and bit more oil to the saucepan, stirring to coat the couscous. Remove the couscous and reserve.

Add broth and oregano to the saucepan and bring to a boil. Reduce the heat to low, stir in couscous and broccoli flowerets. Simmer, covered for 7 minutes.

Stir the softened bell pepper and almonds into couscous. Remove the couscous from heat and set aside, covered, for two more minutes. Serve.

Vegetarian version: Use canned or homemade vegetable broth instead of the chicken broth.

Low-oxalate version: Omit bell pepper, increase broccoli to 4½ cups.

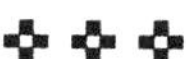

Greek Noodles 

serves 2

¼ lb. angel hair pasta, cooked
2 Tbsp. butter
1 tsp. poppy seed
½ tsp. onion salt

Cook angel hair in boiling water just until tender, but not mushy. Drain and rinse for a few seconds under cold running water. Drain in a colander. Meanwhile, melt butter in a saucepan, being careful not to scorch. Add onion salt and poppy seed. Stir in noodles, working quickly to keep them from sticking to the pan. Serve when noodles are heated through, about two minutes.

When Life Gives You Lemons... Clean Copper

So you've grated the peel for use in foods, now what do you do with the rest of the lemon? Sprinkle salt generously on the cut half of the lemon and rub it on the copper bottom of a saucepan to clean it.

Basmati Rice with Scallops

serves 3

In India, basmati rice is enjoyed for its nut-like aroma. This delicately flavored side dish complements any seafood course.

1 Tbsp. margarine
4 white cardamom pods
¼ c. fresh chives or green onion, chopped
½ c. basmati rice
1⅓ c. water
½ c. green bell pepper, chopped
1 tsp. lemon peel, grated
½ lb. fresh bay scallops
salt to taste

In a heavy saucepan, melt margarine over medium heat and add cardamom pods. Cook a minute or so until pods soften, then press with a fork so the pods crack open, but do not break open completely. Add chives or onions, and cook a minute or so more til soft. Stir in rice, coating with margarine. Add water and bring to a boil.

When boiling, add bell pepper, lemon peel, and scallops, then reduce heat, cover and simmer for 15 minutes. Remove cover and continue to heat over low heat until all water is evaporated. Remove the 4 cardamom pods and serve.

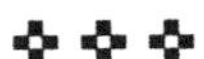

Baked Rice with Peas

serves 3

1⅓ c. low-sodium chicken broth ★
3 Tbsp. margarine or butter
2½ tsp. dried parsley
¾ tsp. garlic powder
½ c. converted white rice
1 c. frozen peas
½ tsp. poppy seed
salt to taste

Preheat oven to 350° F. Bring chicken broth to a boil in a saucepan. Add margarine, parsley and garlic powder. When margarine is melted, remove from heat and add rice, peas, and poppy seed. Turn into a 1½- quart cassserole.

Cover and bake at 350° F. for 40 minutes. Stir and uncover casserole. Bake uncovered for 10 minutes more. Stir in salt if desired and serve. (This dish can be made as a one-dish meal by adding 1 cup cubed, cooked chicken).

MISCELLANEOUS

Low-Acid Blueberry "Jam" ✿

The recipe below makes a delicious spread for toast, and is a variation of the recipe for Homemade Berry Dessert Topping. Not a true jam, it must be kept in the refrigerator, where it will remain fresh for quite awhile.

½ c. sugar
2 Tbsp. flour
1 tsp. Knox unflavored gelatin
¼ tsp. ground cinnamon
2 c. fresh, ripe blueberries
¼ tsp. lemon extract, optional
6 Tbsp. water

Thoroughly mix the sugar, flour, gelatin, and cinnamon in a saucepan. Add blueberries, lemon extract and water. Heat while stirring, coating the blueberries with the sugar. Bring to a boil over medium to high heat, stirring continuously to prevent scorching. Continue stirring and cooking one minute more. Pour into a heat proof container to cool. Store covered in refrigerator until ready to use.

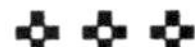

The Ins and Outs of a Jam

A few summers ago, I discovered I could get away with eating a dead-ripe apricot from a neighbor's tree, but not a tablespoon of store-bought apricot jam. This piqued my curiosity. What was it about the jam that set off my bladder? An artificial ingredient?

On my next trip to the market I searched for all-natural, fruit-sweetened jams that didn't list citric acid. Unfortunately, those produced bladder pain too.

I *really* wanted to enjoy jam on my morning toast and became stubbornly determined to do it, one way or another. I went on a jam-making binge. My husband just shook his head, muttering something about pig-headedness.

It was soon obvious that my homemade jam was less likely to rile my bladder than the store-bought kind. Still, it wasn't entirely welcomed by my body. As a last ditch efffort, I tried leaving out the small amount of lemon juice that the recipe called for. Big mistake. Instead of jam, I had a *huge* batch of fruity pancake syrup!

I've learned a few things since then, and now at least I know where I went wrong. Store-bought jams and jellies may be more acid than the ones you make at home because manufacturers will add synthetically produced citric acid to the product both to discourage bacterial growth, and help it set up properly. They are very concerned about product safety, so if anything, they tend to err on the side of too much acidity.

For jams, jellies, or preserves, a certain amount of acidity is necessary to initiate the chemical process involved in turning a liquid into a gel. Citric acid is commonly used in commercial recipes because, unlike some other acids, citric acid is not destroyed by the heat of cooking or processing.

Homemade recipes usually call for lemon juice or orange juice, which are both high in citric acid. Some recipes also call for pectin, a carbohydrate occurring naturally in ripe fruits, to help the process along. (Pectin doesn't seem to bother my bladder).

After a lot of tinkering with fruit concoctions, I've discovered some tasty spreadable low-acid substitutes for traditional jam that can be easily and quickly made at home using fresh fruit. The one drawback is that these lower-acid versions of jams must be stored in the refrigerator. They also need to be used within a short time. They can't be canned, or stored on the shelf as regular jam can.

Try the blueberry recipe in this book, and experiment with any other fruit that you think you may be able to eat. Apricots are a good place to start. Watch out for plums though, because they are acidic as well as naturally high in tyramine. Keep in mind too, that while acidity decreases as fruit ripens, when it becomes over-ripe and spoils, the tyramine content may increase as a result of bacterial action. For the lowest-possible acid and tyramine content, avoid both green and over-ripe fruit.

Coffee, IC-Style

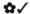

Here's a method of coffee-making which yields a passably good-tasting cup of coffee that is both low in caffeine and low-acid. The idea is to produce a cold concentrate, which is then reconstituted with hot water to make a cup of coffee. Some people can tolerate coffee if it is made this way.

1½ c. ground coffee (ground for a drip coffee maker, see note)
2 c. cold water (see note)
1 quart-size covered container, preferably glass or ceramic
1 half-quart container (also preferably glass or ceramic), which can seal airtight
1 large strainer, colander, or filter holder of a drip-style coffee maker
unbleached paper coffee filters

In a 1-qt. container add the ground coffee to the 2 cups of cold water, stirring to make sure all the coffee is wet. Cover and place in the refrigerator, letting it remain undisturbed for 18 hours.

Remove and uncover. Strain the grounds and liquid through a regular mesh strainer just to get most of the grounds out. (It will be murky with a lot of fine grounds still in the liquid). Then line a strainer, colander or filter holder with a paper coffee filter. Pour or dip out the murky concentrate into the filter paper and let the liquid drip through into another non-plastic container. This may take 30 minutes to an hour, but will produce a concentrate that is clear and sediment-free. (Tip: If you use a coffee-filter holder, make sure there isn't an airtight seal around the area where the filter holder sits on the container. I found out the hard way that the pressure inside the container builds up and it keeps the fluid from being able to drip into the container. You'll wait an awfully long time for the concentrate to drip through). When the coffee concentrate is done, store it in the refrigerator. The recipe above will make about 1 cup of concentrate.

To make a cup of coffee, measure two tablespoons of concentrate (more or less to taste) into a cup or mug. Add ¾ cup boiling water. One cup of the concentrate will make about 8 cups of coffee by this method.

The coffee concentrate can be used in cooking too, if you have a recipe that calls for coffee (try adding a bit to the recipe for Carob Cupcakes, pg. 97).

Note: Be sure to use decaf coffee, and it's a good idea to use coffee ground from low-acid beans. I buy whole coffee beans so I know they are the lowest-acid possible, and grind them myself in a little Krups grinder. A quarter-pound of whole beans (about 1½ cups of whole beans) makes 1½ cups of ground coffee. (See the section on coffee, Part 1).

Try using Evian or another low-acid bottled water. No sense in using low-acid beans then nullifying the effect with acidic water.

Ceramic or glass containers are a good idea for making the concentrate. That way any oils, chemicals, or flavors which may be left in a plastic one don't leach out and ruin the coffee flavor. (The concentrate also stains plastic).

After it is made, it is very important to keep the air out to prevent oxidation and rancidity, as well as to keep your refrigerator from smelling and tasting of coffee. The concentrate will keep for a week or two. Some people freeze the concentrate in ice-cube trays, but I think it loses a bit of flavor that way.

"Sour Cream" Base 

makes ¾ cup

1 c. cottage cheese
6 Tbsp. low-fat milk

Place cottage cheese in a large wire strainer and run cold water over it, washing away the liquid, until water runs clear. Let drain for about ten minutes, then place curds and milk in a blender or food processor and whirl until it is completely smooth.

You'll have to stop every so often to push the mixture onto the blades and test for graininess. It will take about five to seven minutes to do this. One cup of cottage cheese will make about three-quarters of a cup of "sour cream" base. It keeps in the refrigerator as long as cottage cheese does, and is useful in salad dressings or low-fat toppings for baked potatoes. Cottage cheese lacks the acid "bite" of sour cream, so you may want to add a few drops of lemon juice or vinegar, adjusting the level to your bladder's sensitivity.

Sour Cream Substitutes

Although there are some drawbacks to using them, other alternatives (besides the above recipe) exist for sour cream substitutes.

Imitation sour cream products can sometimes be found in supermarkets, and the most popular and reasonably priced brand is "IMO". These products are made with oil, whey, and some fillers like guar gum. They taste fine and work very well in salad dressings, on top of baked potatoes, or as a thickener.

Read the label carefully though. A few IC patients may be bothered by the sodium citrate. The rennet, guar gum or other constituents may also cause a problem for those with irritable bowel syndrome. (Guar gum seems to provoke my IBS symptoms something awful).

Another consideration is fat content. Imitation sour creams are typically made with generous amounts of tropical oils like coconut or palm oil. Not only is imitation sour cream high in fat, a whopping 91% of that fat is artery-clogging *saturated* fat. Even the fat in lard is less saturated. (Some folks with irritable bowel syndrome say foods high in saturated fat trigger symptoms).

Fat Content of Sour Cream and Sour Cream Substitutes

sour cream *(1 cup)*
calories: 490
grams of total fat: 48
percent calories from fat: 86

imitation sour cream *(1 cup)*
calories: 480
grams total fat: 45
percent calories from fat: 83

dry-curd cottage cheese *(1 cup)*
calories: 120
grams total fat: 1
percent calories from fat: 5

Nutritional information from U.S. Dept. of Agriculture, Nutrient Data Laboratory, Food Composition Data (updated Apr. 13, 1997).

Dried Citrus Peel ✿

Citrus peel can add a touch of non-acidic citrus flavor to many foods. It is high in oxalates, so those who have vulvodynia as well as IC may want to avoid it. It is best fresh, but dried peel can work well in a lot of dishes, too. Just remember to use half as much dried peel as fresh. Here's how to make dried citrus peel for later use:

Preheat the oven to 250° F., and while it is heating, finely grate the peel onto a non-stick cookie sheet or an aluminum foil-covered baking sheet. Keep the grated peel spread out, not in one big clump.

Put the cookie sheet in the center of the oven and immediately turn the heat down to 150° F. Let the peel dry in the oven for 1½ to 2 hours or until it is dry and no longer sticky.

Take the sheet out and let the peel air-cool for awhile. When the peel is cool, break up any bits that are stuck together by crushing (a spatula or meat hammer works well). Store in an air-tight container in a dark place. Light, especially ultraviolet light from fluorescent tubes, will cause the peel (and spices too) to lose color and flavor. Brown glass is an excellent way to store the peel. I use large empty brown glass or brown plastic pill containers.

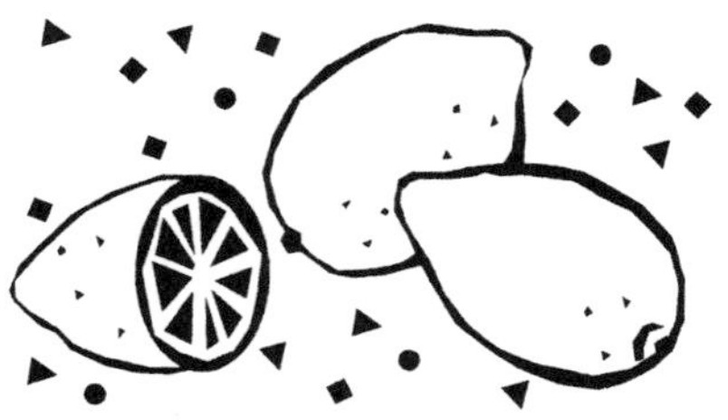

Food-Related Fun: Drying Herbs and Seeds

This may not help your IC symptoms and the product may not be better than similar additive-free items found at specialty stores, but it is an easy and fun activity if you have a garden. You can get some fresh air and exercise. You may even save a little money. But most of all, it's just a creative activity to enjoy alone or as a family project with the kids or grandkids.

Preserving Home-Grown Herbs

There are several ways to dry herbs. They all preserve the essential oils that give the herbs their flavor. The trick is to use very low heat, circulate air, and keep the herbs out of sunlight.

If you live in an area where summers are hot and dry, you can air-dry herbs. To air-dry, first cut the herbs while fresh. Usually, the morning is the best time to do this. Rinse them and tie the stems together with a string. Poke the ends of the stems through a hole cut in the bottom of a paper bag. This way, the bag shields the herbs from direct sunlight, but the bottom is open to allow air to circulate. Hang in a slightly breezy area to dry for a couple of days. As soon as they are dry, store in a tightly capped glass jar in a cool, dark place.

Drying herbs in the oven works well too. Rinse the herbs and lay on a cookie sheet in the center of the oven. Prop the oven door open a bit to let moisture escape. Turn the oven on but don't let the oven temperature exceed 110° F. or the herbs may scorch and flavor will be lost. This may be hard to do with an electric oven, but I've had some success with using an oven thermometer and preheating the oven to about the right temperature, then turning it off while the herbs dry. This requires some attention, since you will have to re-heat the oven a couple of times.

For large-leafed herbs like basil, you can pull the leaves off first, but with the smaller-leafed ones like rosemary, it's easier to do that after they are dried.

A food dehydrator works well to dry herbs too. Be sure to use a temperature setting below 110° F. though.

Herb expert Phyllis Shaudys actually microwaves her herbs to dry them. She says it works for all kinds of herbs, so I tried it with some mint and rosemary I grow in my back yard. Sure enough, it was the quickest and easiest method. Here's how to microwave-dry herbs:

1. Rinse herbs off and dry them.
2. Place them between two layers of paper towels in the microwave.
3. Microwave on high for 30 seconds at a time, keeping note of how long they are being "cooked." Check them to see they aren't getting over-done.
4. Air dry them for a few minutes to allow them to release their remaining moisture. Most herbs take only two or three minutes of microwave time.

Storing in tightly capped containers out of the light is important. Herbs will lose flavor and color as the energy from light changes some of the delicate chemical substances in them. Those decorative little spice shelves meant for hanging on the kitchen wall are really not good for the herbs. The light in your kitchen will deteriorate their quality quickly, especially if you have flourescent lights, or your rack is near a window.

Drying and Roasting Seeds

Kids love to plant sunflowers and watch them grow. (And birds like to eat the seeds if you're not careful!) It's fun and easy to dry and roast sunflower seeds, too.

When the seeds are ripe, allow them to dry on the plant. (Old pantyhose over the seeds may help keep birds away). You can also harvest the seeds and allow them to dry in the sun on a cookie sheet.

Once they are dry, you can salt them before roasting by this method: Soak the sunflower seeds in a solution of two tablespoons of salt to a half a gallon of water. Let them soak overnight or about nine hours. Then remove them and re-dry them for a couple of days.

To roast dried seeds (salted or not), turn your oven to 350° F. Shell the seeds and spread them out on a cookie sheet. Make sure seeds are in a single layer and evenly distributed. Place on a rack in the center of the oven, and roast until they are crisp, about fifteen minutes. Watch them carefully, because they can scorch quickly.

Seeds from a Halloween pumpkins can be roasted too. First remove the seeds from your pumpkin and spread on a cookie sheet. Preheat oven to 120° F., then turn the oven off and put the seeds in. Prop oven door slightly open and let the seeds and fibers dry overnight. (They can also be air-dried for a couple days). When seeds are dry, the fibers can be removed easily.

Shell the pumpkin seeds by removing the hard, white, outer coat. Melt a tablespoon of margarine with half a teaspoon of salt, for each cup of seeds. Toss the shelled seeds with the salt and margarine, then spread seeds on a cookie sheet.

Bake at 325° F. until crisp, which will take about ten or fifteen minutes. Stir them often and keep an eye on them so they don't burn.

Mayonnaise Substitutes ✿

Mayonnaise is one of those commonplace foods that's hard to avoid completely. Butter on sandwiches just isn't the same, and in some recipes there's no handy substitute that people with IC can use. Commercially prepared mayonnaise products have two problems to watch out for: additives such as MSG (listed on the label or not), and acidity. (See Appendix B for additive-free mayonnaise products your bladder may tolerate). If acidity is the main problem for you, try this recipe for acid-free mayonnaise. If this recipe still gives you bladder problems, try making it without the spices.

2 c. salad oil, divided

½ tsp. dry mustard

½ tsp. salt

dash ground black pepper

2 egg yolks

¼ tsp. lemon extract

2 Tbsp. water

Pour ¼ cup of the salad oil in a small dish and pour 1¾ cups of oil in another. Set aside. In a small bowl, combine the mustard, salt, and pepper. Add egg yolks and beat with electric mixer until blended. Add the oil *one teaspoon at a time*, from the dish with the quarter-cup of oil, while beating constantly. When that is gone, add the rest of the oil in a thin, steady, stream while continuing to beat. Beat in lemon extract and water last. Store refrigerated in an airtight container up to 4 weeks.

PART THREE

APPENDIX A

Some Notes on Dietary Supplements

If you are like a lot of people with IC, you've no doubt tried vitamins and other nutritional dietary supplements. Taking a few pills each morning seems to be an easy way to make sure you're getting what your body needs. And don't we all secretly hope that if our bodies just get all the right vitamins and minerals, maybe the IC will disappear? Unfortunately, some of us have found out the hard way that certain vitamin supplements can even make our bladder symptoms worse.

Vitamins and minerals

Although some people have had good experiences with vitamins, there are a few things to watch out for. It appears that one problem is the acidic form of vitamin preparations. Vitamin C, for instance, is usually found in the form of ascorbic acid. Many people with IC cannot tolerate this acidic vitamin preparation, yet it is by far the most common way it is sold. Although some of us can't take ascorbic acid at all, others can take it if the acidity is buffered. The usual buffering agent is calcium carbonate, the major ingredient of Tums. Another vitamin C preparation on the market is "Ester-C." Some can tolerate this form, but often people with severe IC pain can't take this form either.

Vitamin B-6 is another problematic vitamin supplement. It is usually sold in the form of pyridoxine hydrochloride. Pyridoxine hydrochloride is notorious among IC sufferers for causing bladder symptom flares. There are actually three forms of vitamin B-6. In rats, the three forms are equally active, and scientists have assumed that it works that way in people too. It is very difficult however, to find commercially produced vitamin B-6 in forms other than pyridoxine hydrochloride.

Magnesium is another dietary supplement that has caused problems for some IC sufferers, particularly those who have the constipation-type irritable bowel syndrome, or take constipating pain medications. This is an interesting phenomenon, because magnesium preparations generally have a laxative effect for most people. Too much of an iron supplement or calcium carbonate can also have a constipating effect.

Another interesting phenomenon is that although some vitamin supplements cause IC symptom flares, the same amount of those vitamins when found in food appear not to have the effect. The daily requirement of vitamins C and B-6 can be obtained by consuming bladder-friendly foods. For example, which do you think has more vitamin C, oranges or bell peppers? Bell peppers are actually higher in vitamin C, although most people think of oranges as being "the vitamin-C food." We can get an adequate intake of vitamin C by eating bell peppers and other vegetables.

Vitamin B-6 is a little harder to get because foods that contain significant amounts of it are limited, and because it is sensitive to heat. Cooking or processing food can destroy up to 50% of it. More than 75% of the B-6 in wheat is lost during the milling of white flour. The good news is, several bladder-friendly foods are high in vitamin B-6. Cashews, almonds, and especially sunflower seeds are good, natural, bladder-friendly sources of B-6, and make a delicious snack. (Watch out for artificial ingredients, hot spices, sulfites, hydrolyzed vegetable protein, or MSG on the seeds and nuts. Read the labels carefully).

Some IC patients have favorite vitamin or mineral products which they take daily, and which seem to cause them no difficulty. Although many are simply taking the supplements for general purposes and haven't felt any improvement in their IC, others have very positive experiences to report. Here is one person's story: An IC patient on Elmiron, who was suffering hair loss as a side effect, wrote a plea for help and posted it on an internet newsgroup. Another woman named Carole, posted a reply about her own hair loss experience, saying, "I recommend biotin, 500 mcg. per day, to minimize hair loss. It works for me and for some other people I know... I'd take it even if I wasn't taking Elmiron, simply because of how healthy my hair is since I started taking it."

Be sure to consult your doctor about taking dietary supplements though, because some may interact unfavorably with certain medications. Watch out too, for artificial ingredients, fillers and preservatives in some of the preparations— some of which may not appear on the label.

Bioflavonoids and antioxidants

Bioflavonoids are biologically active compounds of a chemical class known as flavonoids. These compounds are found in fruits, berries, and various plant products. In plants, they often exist in combination with vitamin C. Some bioflavonoids are available as dietary supplements in health food stores and a few grocery stores (usually in the antioxidant section).

The role that bioflavonoids play in the human body is only beginning to be understood, yet what is known so far about this class of chemicals is intriguing. One area that has attracted scientific attention is the possible effect of bioflavonoids on capillary fragility. Capillaries which easily break and bleed into the skin (evidenced by little pinpoint red spots under the skin) are a sign of capillary fragility. Bioflavonoids appear to have an influence on capillary fragility and some authorities speculate that because bioflavonoids are found together in nature with vitamin C, that they may function with vitamin C to increase the strength of capillaries and regulate their permeability to fluids. That line of reasoning has led many manufacturers to combine bioflavonoids with vitamin C in their products.

Many claims for the bioflavonoid products sold at health food stores can be found in holistic publications. Boosters of these products proclaim wide-ranging (and often absurdly inflated) health benefits which have not been scientifically proven. Nonetheless, if you want to get more bioflavonoids in your diet, eating fruits and vegetables may be the most practical and inexpensive way. Bioflavonoids are not easily damaged by processing or cooking, and losses due to lengthy storage are also small (as long as they aren't exposed to strong light). Foods like red bell peppers, broccoli, and even cooked red onions, can be excellent sources of bioflavonoids.

Many bioflavonoids function as antioxidants. Antioxidants are another area of intense scientific investigation. Many plants appear to contain compounds, called antioxidants, which can mop up or destroy free radicals. These free radicals are substances which can cause cellular damage, even cancer, in humans. Our own bodies produce free radicals as a by-product of normal activity, and we also have mechanisms to clear the body of free radicals. However, scientists are suspecting that the antioxidants in fruits and vegetables may be important in helping our bodies get rid of free radicals. Based on the scientific evidence to date, the U.C. Berkeley School of Public Health, in advice to the general public concerning antioxidants, recommends eating "at least five antioxidant-rich fruits and vegetables daily."

The dietary supplement pycnogenol is an extract derived from the French maritime pine, *pinus maritima*. It has been used by doctors in Europe for many years to treat such things as varicose veins and the poor circulation associated with diabetes. Discovered and patented by Jacques Masquelier of the University of Quebec, it contains over forty polyphenols and phytochemicals. Dr. Lester Packer, a researcher at the University of California, Berkeley, is one of many scientists interested in pycnogenol's antioxidant properties, though he admits that scientific understanding of its effects is limited.

There is much hype in the holistic press concerning pycnogenol's health benefits, although according to the FDA, there is no proof that it is helpful in treating any disease. Despite this, there are some people with IC who say that taking it has helped their IC pain and frequency. In the winter 1996 issue of the *ICA Update*, urologist and IC researcher Dr. Kristene Whitmore reports some of her IC patients' positive experiences, saying, "Herbal immune stimulants such as echinacea, ginseng, pycnogenol (pine bark which acts as an immune stimulant) and co-enzyme Q10 (another immune stimulant) have been found to be useful by some people."

A few years ago, I and a group of regulars at an IC support group tried pine-bark pycnogenol for our IC symptoms. After several months of daily doses of pycnogenol, it seemed that some of us benefitted a little, others said it did nothing, while a couple of people claimed it practically vanquished their symptoms. We all found it to be quite expensive, though. To save money, some of us switched to the grape-seed extract (also sold in health food stores as "pycnogenol"). Though cheaper, one of the ladies whose urinary frequency had improved on the pine-bark extract, reported that the grape-seed extract did nothing for her. Over several months I found the pine bark pycnogenol did seem to help my pain somewhat, but I decided that for me at least, the minor amount of pain relief wasn't worth the major expense.

Amino acids and IC

Amino acids are the building blocks of protein, so when we eat foods with protein (and even vegetables contain proteins), we take in amino acids. Some amino acids are considered "essential," which means our body does not make them. Others are both manufactured by the body and are available from food. Several amino acids are worth mentioning, because they may have an effect on IC symptoms.

First is the amino acid, histidine. Sold as a dietary supplement in health food stores, it is a constituent of certain protein health food products. It can be converted in the body to histamine, that noxious substance that triggers mast cells and causes inflammation. Be very careful to read labels. I had a bad experience once when I tried a protein powder drink which, unbeknownst to me, contained a large amount of histidine. I will never forget the excruciating pain that resulted.

In April 1996, researchers at Yale reported in *The Journal of Urology* that IC patients have a deficiency in an enzyme that synthesizes nitric oxide. Nitric oxide is a small molecule, the tiniest that the body manufactures. But it is very important in a number of bodily functions, including the regulation of blood flow. (In the intestinal tract, irritable bowel syndrome has been linked to nitric oxide's action, and in the bladder it is thought to be significant as well). Dr. Shannon Smith and the others at Yale suspected that the bladder pain and spasms associated with IC may be the result of impaired blood circulation in the bladder. They wondered if the amino acid arginine, which the body uses to produce nitric oxide, could help.

They tested their hypothesis on a handful of IC patients, and the rest is history—the effects of taking arginine supplements were positive and dramatic. As soon as the results were announced in the *ICA Update*, many people with IC rushed out to their local health food stores to buy the dietary supplement, L-arginine, and try it for themselves. (The "L" refers to the shape of the molecule. Arginine comes in two shapes which, like your right and left hands, are mirror images of each other). Although it doesn't help everyone, some people find it relieves bladder pain. It helps me somewhat with the aching and general abdominal tenderness associated with IC. If you want to try L-arginine, ask your doctor about dosage and possible drug interactions.

I feel that one other amino acid is worth mentioning, mostly due to my own bad experience with it. That amino acid is lysine. Many people that suffer from genital herpes, Chronic Fatigue Syndrome (CFS) or fever blisters treat them by taking L-lysine dietary supplements. Several articles have appeared in popular magazines concerning the beneficial effects of L-lysine. In December 1995, after one such article hit the newsstand, three IC sufferers who frequented an internet IC message board, including myself, all decided to try L-lysine on the idea that perhaps IC was caused by a virus. Since L-lysine dietary supplements had helped one man with CFS and another with herpes simplex outbreaks, according to a *Saturday Evening Post* article, we figured perhaps lysine might help us too. After all, we were tired all the time too, and who knows, there might be a viral connection to IC. I purchased a bottle of L-lysine at a nearby health food store and began by taking just one capsule a day. Within a couple of days I was having a terrible flare of bladder pain. I stopped the L-lysine, and the flare stopped. I started the L-lysine again, and sure enough, I had more excruciating bladder pain. I was certain the L-lysine was at fault but couldn't figure out why. The two other women trying L-lysine supplements soon posted messages on the internet IC board saying that it either made their bladder symptoms worse, or did nothing at all to help.

I looked at the *Post* articles again. One of them mentioned that lysine competes with receptors for arginine in the body, and the article went on to advise those with fever blisters to avoid foods high in arginine. It listed several foods high in arginine and low in lysine, including these IC-friendly foods: almonds, white rice, popcorn, sunflower seeds and coconut. Hmm, I thought, could arginine help if lysine hurt? By the time I had the idea to try L-arginine supplements, Dr. Smith's findings on arginine were surfacing in the IC patient community, and a possible reason for my lysine-induced bladder symptom flare became apparent.

Nutrients in food

Many doctors hold the view that eating fruits and vegetables is the most sensible way to get antioxidants and other nutrients. After all, they say, man has evolved for millions of years and during that period he has been eating vitamins, minerals, amino acids, and antioxidants in combination with other substances in foods, not alone in pill form. It would make sense that our bodies are designed to take in and utilize these substances, not alone, but in combination with the thousands of other substances in the foods we eat. One interesting experiment that supports this notion found that certain antioxidant vitamins neutralized free radicals much better when they were in foods, than they did when working alone.

Effects of food storage and preparation

The old saying "less is more" certainly applies to food storage. The less time you store foods, especially fresh vegetables and fruits, the more vitamins are maintained. For vegetables, the amount of wilting is a good rule-of-thumb indicator of the amount of vitamin loss during storage. Buying the freshest produce available can help increase the nutritive value of your diet. But don't throw away those canned veggies. According to the November 1997 issue of the *University of California Berkeley Wellness Letter*, a newsletter of the School of Public Health, "Nine out of ten people believe that fresh vegetables are more nutritious than frozen or canned, but this is often not the case, unless the fresh items are really fresh. Nutrients are more or less 'locked in' when produce is frozen or canned."

With eggs, refrigeration is very important because, despite their protective shell, they can become contaminated when left at room temperature for long periods. First, be sure to always buy refrigerated eggs. Occasionally stores may promote egg sales by stacking cartons in the aisles, unrefrigerated. This dangerous practice can increase spoilage of the eggs and may be responsible for some cases of salmonella. Cooking well makes sure that infective organisms are killed.

One of the amino acids which make up the protein we eat, tyrosine, can be converted to tyramine, a substance suspected of triggering IC symptoms. Micro-organisms commonly found in food can do the conversion job. If your bladder is extremely sensitive to the effects of tyramine in food, you may want to take special care that all protein foods (meats, eggs, milk, fish, casseroles, etc.) are properly refrigerated or stored, and that they are eaten promptly. Here is one bad experience I had with some Muenster cheese (which usually doesn't bother my bladder): I bought a large piece at the store, making sure it was fresh. When I got it home, I used some for topping a casserole then refrigerated the rest. The leftover cheese got pushed to the back of the refrigerator and went unnoticed for a couple of weeks. Then one evening while scrounging for snacks, I noticed the cheese. I checked it for mold, and finding none, I snacked on a small slice. Within hours I was having horrible stabbing pains in my bladder and urethra. But it's not just protein foods that can become high in tyramine. According to nutrition expert Susan G. Dudek, writing in *The Nutrition Handbook of Nursing Practice* (Lipincott-Raven, 3rd ed., 1997), spoiled and overripe fruit can become high in tyramine too.

Sodium and Potassium

There is some confusion in the patient community regarding the role of dietary sodium and potassium, and whether or not one should modify their intake. Comments by certain prominent IC researchers have spurred scientific debate over the effects of sodium and potassium ions on the IC bladder, but have also served to confuse patients even more. Rather than get involved in a debate whose merits I'm not qualified to judge, I'll just present a few basic facts here. Once again, as with so many things about IC, this may be an area where individuals vary. If you experiment with your diet and feel that your sodium or potassium intake may exacerbate your symptoms, it is important to talk to your doctor before making drastic dietary changes.

We are all familiar with the effect of putting salt on an open skin wound such as a knee abrasion— it burns and stings. Yet if we eat a salty pretzel when we have a skinned knee, we don't experience the same burning and stinging at our wound. Salt (sodium chloride) makes the wound burn when applied directly because the salt's ions stimulate raw nerve endings in the skin. But when we eat salt, the sodium and chlorine ions become part of a complex web of chemical interactions in our body, and we don't necessarily have the same physical reaction as if we applied it directly to raw skin.

Potassium can cause reactions in nerves and muscle tissue similar to sodium. Like table salt, when potassium salt (sold as salt substitute in stores) is applied to an exposed muscle, the muscle will contract. Likewise, when we eat foods with potassium or potassium salts, they affect many bodily systems and we won't get the same results as we would if we merely sprinkled some on a wound.

It has been noted by IC researcher Dr. Lowell Parsons that certain potassium compounds can cause pain and urgency when instilled in some people's "leaky" IC bladders, whereas healthy volunteers feel nothing. At his clinic in San Diego, Dr. Parsons uses a potassium solution to help distinguish which IC patients have "leaky" bladders— bladder linings that allow the potassium salt solution to "leak" through to the bladder's muscle tissue. Interestingly, while some sodium and potassium compounds can cause pain when instilled in IC bladders, other sodium-containing compounds such as sodium pentosan polysulfate (Elmiron) or heparin sodium actually soothe the IC bladder. Dr. Parsons, in an interview published in the ICA *Update* (Fall 1996, Vol. 11, #3, pages 4-5), advocates oral doses of potassium citrate (a urinary alkalinizer) as beneficial for some IC patients. He comments, "There are no real side effects except possibly gastrointestinal (nausea or loose stools) when you take it, but these effects do not occur at the lower doses in most patients. I recommend using two doses per day which can be quite beneficial." Unfortunately, while some are helped by oral potassium citrate, others find it causes flares. As with so many other things, each IC patient is different.

So what about high-potassium and high-sodium foods? In general do they help or harm with regard to bladder pain? While no clinical experiments have been done on people with IC, we can look to the laboratory of life and do a "reality check" via our own experiences. High-potassium foods don't seem to have any effect my bladder. I asked a few of my friends who have IC if they'd noticed anything about salty food, or food high in potassium. They all said they hadn't been aware of any problem. If you'd like to do your own check, here are some typical levels of potassium found in 100 grams (about 3½ ounces) of some common "IC-safe" foods, according to the USDA's Nutrient Database: blanched almonds, 750 mg.; beef (cooked, round), 392 mg.; chicken (cooked), 243 mg.; pear, 125 mg.; blueberries, 89 mg. And here are some typical levels of potassium in 100 grams of some "IC-pain provokers:" banana, 396 mg.; yogurt (from skim milk), 255 mg.; navel orange, 178 mg.; cranberries, 71 mg.

Levels of sodium are listed on food labels so you can easily find out if there is any relation to your IC flares. Cottage cheese or salted french fries (both high in sodium) don't cause my bladder pain to increase, and baking soda actually helps— but you may be different. Lisa, for instance, cannot tolerate calcium carbonate, a substance that helps most IC patients with their bladder pain.

There is one thing that many with IC have noted, and which may bear on this issue. When I get dehydrated, my IC pain is worse. Karen experiences the same thing. She says, "I have to make sure I drink enough water or I'm in real trouble. It's not easy if I'm busy or out shopping, but if I think I may not drink enough, I'll take water with me." Sharon speculates her pain may be related to the "saltiness" of her urine. "I think my bladder is really sensitive to salty urine, so I try to dilute it by drinking water when I can."

Nutrients and What They Do

With any diet that restricts the intake of so many foods comes the worry, "Am I getting proper nutrition? Am I getting all the vitamins I need?" I can't answer that question for you, but it isn't very difficult to get all the vitamins doctors say is normally required for good all-around nutrition, and still stick to your IC diet. Here is a list of some major nutrients, along with some IC-friendly foods that are sources of that nutrient. If you want more detailed information, or would like professional meal-planning guidance, consult a registered dietician. Your doctor or the American Dietetic Association (see Appendix C, pg. 221) can help you locate one.

NUTRIENT	SOME FUNCTIONS	GOOD FOOD SOURCES
Biotin	Essential to metabolize carbohydrates, proteins, and fats.	Cauliflower, nuts (ie., cashews, almonds), egg yolk. (Also made by microorganisms in the gastrointestinal tract).
Calcium	Necessary for maintaining bones and teeth. Blood clotting, muscle contraction and relaxation, cell wall permeability, and nerve function.	Milk, milk products (ie., cream cheese, whipped cream, cottage cheese, ricotta), green leafy vegetables, fish and cereal products (ie., corn, wheat, rice, oat, barley, soy).
Carbohydrate	Supplies energy, and some sources also provide fiber.	Bread and cereal products made from whole grains, starchy vegetables (ie., potatoes), fruits (ie., pears and blueberries), sugars.
Chlorine	Helps regulate acid-base balance and water balance. Needed to form stomach acid and involved in absorption of vitamin B-12 and iron.	Salt and foods containing salt.

Chromium	Stabilizes nucleic acids, activates enzymes, and is a component of GTF (glucose tolerance factor), which enhances the effect of insulin.	Many fresh foods, especially beef, eggs, and oysters.
Cobalt	Important in forming vitamin B-12.	Green leafy vegetables (ie., cabbage, spinach, lettuce).
Copper	Helps form important proteins and hemoglobin. Aids in bone formation.	Nuts (ie., cashews, almonds) and seeds, oysters, whole-grain cereal products (ie., cornbread, whole wheat bread).
Fats	Provide food energy and essential fatty acids. Needed to carry fat-soluble vitamins and for regulatory functions.	Vegetable oils, butter, whole milk, cream. margarine, sunflower seeds, nuts (ie., cashews and almonds), and meat fat.
Fluorine	Involved in making strong bones and teeth.	Fluoridated water, shrimp, fish, shellfish.
Folacin (folic acid)	Important for cell division and reproduction, and in the manufacture of hemoglobin.	Green leafy vegetables, pears, blueberries.
Iodine	Essential part of thyroid hormones.	Iodized table salt, kelp, seafood.
Iron	Necessary in formation of hemoglobin in red blood cells, also for enzymes involved in energy metabolism.	Oysters and clams, pork, beef, dried peas and beans, lentils, iron-fortified products. In many fresh foods (except dairy).
Magnesium	Essential part of bones and teeth. Important in nerve function.	Nuts (ie., cashews and almonds), fish, shellfish, whole-grain cereals (ie., wheat, rice, corn, oats).
Manganese	Growth of connective tissue, formation of bone, possibly hair growth.	Whole-grain cereals, green leafy vegetables.

Molybdenum	Component of tooth enamel and of enzymes that metabolize fats and proteins.	Leafy vegetables, legumes (ie., lentils), whole grains.
Niacin (nicotinic acid)	Helps metabolize carbohydrates.	Fish, beef, pork, chicken, lamb, dried peas and beans, lentils.
Pantothenic acid	Part of two enzymes that are important in nerve impulses, hemoglobin formation, synthesis of steroids, and formation of antibodies.	Wheat bran, rice bran, nuts (ie., cashews , almonds), eggs, salmon, brown rice, sunflower seeds.
Phosphorus	Forms and maintains bone and teeth, builds muscles. Involved in many metabolic functions, energy production, and in maintaining acid-base balance.	Milk, milk products (ie., cream cheese, whipped cream, cottage cheese, ricotta), beef, lamb, pork, poultry, fish, nuts (ie., cashews and almonds), whole grains (ie., rice, corn, wheat, oats, barley).
Potassium	Involved in nerve transmission, acid-base balance, and is required for carbohydrate metabolism and protein synthesis. Helps transfer nutrients in and out of individual cells.	Milk, fruit (ie., pears, honeydew, blueberries, raisins), most fresh foods.
Protein	Necessary for formation of new tissues, also in maintenance and regulatory functions.	Meat, fish, poultry, eggs, dried beans, peas, lentils, nuts (ie., cashews and almonds), milk.
Selenium	Interrelated with Vitamin E as an antioxidant, needed to form the enzyme glutathione peroxidase.	Meat, fish, eggs, shrimp, lobster, clams, oysters and other shellfish. Amount in soil influences amount in plant sources.

Sodium	Component of bile and pancreatic juice, associated with muscle contraction and nerve function. Helps maintain water balance and balance of acids and bases in fluids outside of cells.	Salt, snack foods, beef, pork, cornbread, and most fresh foods.
Vitamin A	Necessary for resistance to infection and night vision.	Dark-green leafy vegetables, salmon, oysters, crab, halibut, swordfish, butter, cream.
Vitamin B-1 (thiamine)	Muscle tone, healthy nerves, normal appetite, and energy metabolism.	Lean pork, potatoes, dried peas and beans, nuts (ie., cashews, almonds), whole-grain breads.
Vitamin B-2 (riboflavin)	Metabolizes amino acids and carbohydrates, forms niacin.	Eggs, lean meat, enriched breads, milk.
Vitamin B-6 (pyridoxine)	Involved in protein, carbohydrate and fat metabolism, functioning of central nervous system.	Fish, legumes (ie., dried peas and beans, lentils), whole-grain breads.
Vitamin B-12	Necessary for production of red blood cells, and healthy nerves. Involved in DNA synthesis.	Fish, egg, muscle meats (ie., beef, chicken, lamb, pork), milk. (Most grains and vegetables contain little or none).
Vitamin C	Needed for formation of collagen, absorption of iron, and strong capillary walls and blood vessels. Important in wound healing.	Green bell peppers, potatoes, and green leafy vegetables (ie., cabbage, spinach, lettuce).
Vitamin D	Essential for strong bones and teeth. Needed for calcium and phosphorus absorption.	Egg yolk, butter, cream, milk that has been fortified with vitamin D.

Vitamin E	An antioxidant, it protects essential fatty acids from oxidative destruction. Acts with selenium.	Wheat germ, vegetable oil, margarine, egg yolk, green leafy vegetables, legumes (ie., dried peas and beans, lentils).
Vitamin K	Needed for blood clotting.	Green leafy vegetables, vegetable oils, pork. (Also produced by organisms in the intestine).
Zinc	Component of many enzymes involved in energy metabolism and making proteins, needed for normal skin, bones, and hair. Involved in wound healing.	Most fresh foods, especially vegetables.

Nutritional information:

The Merck Manual, 16th edition. 1992. Edited by Robert Berkow, M.D., Andrew J. Fletcher, M.D., et al., Merck & Co., Inc.

Foods and Nutrition Encyclopedia. 1983. Edited by A.H. Ensminger, M.E. Ensminger, J.E. Konlande, and J.R.K. Robson, M.D., Pegus Press.

APPENDIX B

The IC Pantry

One thing I really loathe doing is having to give up eating one of my cherished recipes because it causes bladder pain. I can still enjoy many of those favorite dishes though, if I substitute IC-friendly versions of certain ingredients for the less-safe ones called for in the recipe. Here are some products that various IC patients have found are more "bladder friendly" than other comparable brands of the same product. Some are national brands, and some are local.

You'll notice that even water is listed. Believe it or not, many people report that plain tap water causes symptom flares. Some claim it is the chlorine— they reduce symptoms by drinking only unchlorinated well water. Others claim their tap water is so acid that they find it helpful to consume only low-acid bottled water. (You can call your local water district and find out if you have very acid or very alkaline water). For bottled water, the acidity may be reported on the label, or it may be disguised in chemical terminology. Acidity is often reported as "pH" followed by a number— and the lower the number, the more acid the water is. Compare labels. I've tried various bottled waters and found some brands are definitely better than others at keeping my bladder happy.

Everyone has different levels of sensitivity, so this list is just a guide. If the suggestions here don't work for you, don't be afraid to experiment with various brands on the market to see what suits your needs. Companies often change formulations too, so it's advisable to check labels now and then, even on products you've used for a long time.

For this Ingredient:	Try Using:
apple juice	Allen's (in Canada) makes a lower-acid apple juice.
bacon bits or Bac-O's	Fakin' Bacon Bits by Lightlife (100% vegetarian, has no artificial ingredients, no MSG).
beef base or beef bouillon cubes	Chef Piero (most brands list MSG, this brand doesn't); Superior Touch "Better Than Bouillon" Beef Base (has hydrolyzed soy protein, but no MSG listed).
beef broth	Health Valley Fat-Free Beef Flavored Broth (has no added MSG).

butterscotch baking morsels	Nestle Butterscotch chips.
chicken broth	Health Valley 100% Natural Chicken Broth (unlike many others, this has no MSG).
chicken broth, low-sodium	Campbell's Healthy Request Chicken Broth or Campbell's Low-sodium Chicken Broth.
chow mein noodles	Chun King.
chopped clams, clam juice	Snow's (unlike many brands, doesn't have MSG).
cloves (spice)	Allspice can often substitute for the more bladder-irritating spice, cloves, in many recipes.
coconut, shredded unsweetened	Whole Foods Brand (has no sulfites or artificial ingredients).
creamed corn	Del Monte No-salt Added cream-style corn.
cream of mushroom soup	Campbell's Healthy Request Cream of Mushroom soup.
dates, chopped	Whole Foods brand (no sulfites), Hadley's (no preservatives).
graham crackers	Keebler Honey Graham Selects (lacks artificial ingredients of other brands. Best for making crumb crusts, too).
jam or jelly	Sorrell Ridge 100% Fruit, wild blueberry; Braswell's Pear Preserves (low-oxalate safe). (Call Braswell's at (912) 764-6191 or fax (912) 489-1572 for a mail order form & product list. View their website: http://www.braswells.com. The pear preserves have such small amount of citric acid that three ladies with severe IC & vulvodynia found it safe).
lemon juice	Grated lemon peel or lemon extract works fine in some recipes.
lime juice	Same as for lemon juice.
mayonnaise	Whole Foods brand (no MSG).
orange juice	Low- or reduced-acid versions of orange juices (Minute Maid makes one); orange peel or extract also works in some recipes.

parsley (fresh or dried)	For those avoiding parsley's high-oxalate content, chervil may be a substitute worth trying.
peanut butter	Laura Scudder's All-Natural Old-Fashioned.
pretzel sticks, pretzels	Von's Fat-free; Snyder's of Hanover Olde Tyme Pretzels.
snack crackers, high fiber	Pepperidge Farm Hearty Wheat, Kavli Crispbread, Nabisco Wheat Thins, Hain Rich Crackers, Ak-mak 100% whole wheat stone-ground sesame crackers, Nabisco Triscuits "original" only. (The company changes formulations often and several versions of this cracker are marketed. Check the label).
snack crackers, low fiber	Carr's Table Water Crackers.
sour cream	I.M.O. works for some people, but high in fat. Some with IBS may also experience problems with some of the ingredients. (See recipe in Part Two, Miscellaneous section).
soy sauce	Chun King Lite (low-sodium).
tomato paste	Contadina tomato paste (although tomato paste in general has problems, at least this one has no MSG).
vanilla ice cream	Dreyer's Grand vanilla ice cream or Edy's vanilla ice cream. Rice Dream (vanilla), and Rice Dream Bars (carob coated).
vegetable beef soup	Campbell's condensed Healthy Request Vegetable made with beef stock, and Campbell's Ready to Serve Low Sodium Chunky Vegetable Beef. (These brands seem tolerable for many people despite small amounts of yeast extract or oleoresin paprika, but be careful if your bladder is very sensitive. You can write to Campbell's for a list of their MSG-free products).
vegetable broth	Health Valley vegetable broth.
water	Evian (nationally), Deer Park (in New York).
white chocolate baking morsels	Ghiradelli white morsels (less artificial ingredients than Nestle's).
yellow food coloring	Turmeric, a slightly sweet, delicately flavored spice that will turn strong tasting food yellow without noticeably affecting the flavor.

Sources for Hard to Find Food Items

We all can relate to the frustration of searching for a hard to find food item at several grocery stores. Here is a list of stores that carry a lot of "natural" grocery products, from preservative-free cereals to gluten-free bread. If your local grocery store doesn't carry an item from the IC Pantry, check these stores. Most likely they will have it, and if not, some of these stores may even order it for you. One word of warning: you will pay more for less. "Natural" products without additives or preservatives tend to spoil more quickly. The store ends up throwing out a lot and that costs them. They pass it along to you in the form of higher prices. Sometimes though, it's worth the cost to find a "safer" version of a favorite food.

These are only *some* of the larger, good quality "chain" stores. These chains are constantly adding new locations and changing store names, so be sure to check you local phone book for some of the company names listed here. Your phone book may also list smaller independent stores that carry many of the same products and are well worth a visit too.

ARIZONA

Wild Oats Community Market

Phoenix (3933 E. Camelback Rd.)	(602) 954-0584
Scottsdale (7129 E. Shea)	(602) 905-1441

Whole Foods Market

Tempe (5120 S. Rural)	(818) 762-5548

CALIFORNIA

Mothers Market & Kitchen

Costa Mesa (225 E. 17th Street)	(714) 631-4741
Huntington Beach (19770 Beach Blvd.)	(714) 963-6667
Irvine (2963 Michelson Dr.)	(714) 752-6667

Whole Foods Market

Berkeley (3000 Telegraph Ave.)	(510) 649-1333
Beverly Hills (239 N. Crescent Dr.)	(310) 274-3360
Campbell (1690 S. Bascom Ave.)	(408) 371-5000
Cupertino (20830 Stevens Creek Blvd.)	(408) 257-7000
Glendale (826 North Glendale Ave.)	(818) 240-9350
La Jolla (8825 La Jolla Dr.)	(619) 642-6700
Los Angeles (11666 National Blvd.)	(310) 996-8840
Los Gatos (15980 Los Gatos Blvd.)	(408) 358-4434

Mill Valley (414 Miller Ave.)	(415) 381-1200
Northridge (9350 Reseda Blvd.)	(818) 701-5122
Palo Alto (774 Emerson St.)	(415) 326-8676
Pacific Grove (173 Central Ave.)	(408) 647-2153
Redondo Beach (405 N. Pacific Coast Hwy.)	(310) 376-6931
San Diego (711 University Ave.)	(619) 294-2800
San Francisco (1765 California St.)	(415) 674-0500
San Rafael (340 Third St.)	(415) 451-6333
Sherman Oaks (12905 Riverside Dr.)	(818) 762-5548
Thousand Oaks (451 Avenida de los Arboles)	(805) 492-5340
Tustin (14945 Holt Ave.)	(714) 731-3400

Wild Oats Community Market

Berkeley (1581 University Ave.)	(510) 549-1714
Laguna Beach (283 Broadway)	(949) 376-7888
Mission Viejo (27142 La Paz Rd.)	(949) 460-0202
Pasadena (603 South Lake Ave.)	(626) 792-1778
Sacramento (5104 Arden Way)	(916) 481-1955
San Anselmo (222 Greenfield Ave.)	(415) 258-0660
Santa Monica (1425 Montana Ave.)	(310) 576-4707
Sunnyvale (1265 S. Mary St.)	(408) 730-1310
West Hollywood (8611 Santa Monica Blvd.)	(310) 854-6927
West Los Angeles (3474 Centinela Ave.)	(310) 636-1300

COLORADO

Alfalfa's

Denver (201 University)	(303) 320-9071
Denver (900 East 11th Ave.)	(303) 832-7701
Lakewood (14357 W. Colfax Ave.)	(303) 277-1339
Littleton (5910 S. University)	(303) 798-9699

Wild Oats Community Market

Aurora (12131 East Iliff Ave.)	(303) 695-8801
Denver (2260 Colfax Ave.)	(303) 320-1664
Denver (1111 So. Washington)	(303) 733-6201
Greenwood Village (6000 S. Holly)	(303) 796-0996
Westminster (9229 N. Sheridan Blvd.)	(303) 650-2333

CONNECTICUT

Fresh Fields

Greenwich (90 E. Putnam Ave.)	(203) 661-0631

FLORIDA

Whole Foods Market

No. Miami Beach (3565 NE 207th Street) (305) 933-1543

Wild Oats Community Market

Boca Raton (2200 West Glades Rd.) (561) 392-5100

Ft. Lauderdale (2501 E. Sunrise Blvd.) (954) 566-9333

West Palm Beach (7735 Dixie Hwy.) (561) 585-8800

ILLINOIS

Fresh Fields

Palatine (1331 North Rand Rd.) (847) 776-8080

Whole Foods Market

Chicago (3300 N. Ashland) (312) 244-4200

Chicago (1000 West North Avenue) (312) 587-0648

Evanston (1640 Chicago Ave.) (847) 733-1600

River Forest (7245 Lake St.) (708) 366-1045

Wheaton (151 Rice Lake Square.) (630) 588-1500

Wild Oats Community Market

Buffalo Grove (764 Buffalo Grove Rd.) (847) 419-9080

KANSAS

Wild Oats Community Market

Mission (5101 Johnson Dr.) (913) 722-4069

LOUISIANA

Whole Foods Market

New Orleans (3135 Esplanade) (504) 943-1626

MARYLAND

Fresh Fields

Annapolis (2504 Solomons Island Rd.) (410) 573-1800

Bethesda (5269 River Rd.) (301) 984-4860

Rockville (1649 Rockville Pk.) (301) 984-4880

MASSACHUSETTS

Bread & Circus

Boston (15 Westland Ave.) (617) 375-1010

Brookline (15 Washington St.) (617) 738-8187

Cambridge (115 Prospect St.)	(617) 492-0070
Cambridge (200 Alewife Brook Pkwy.)	(617) 491-0040
Hadley (Route 9/Russell St.)	(413) 586-9932
Newton (916 Walnut St.)	(617) 969-1141
Wellesley Hills (278 Washington St.)	(781) 235-7262

MICHIGAN

Whole Foods Market

Ann Arbor (2398 E. Stadium Blvd.)	(313) 971-3366

MINNESOTA

Whole Foods Market

St. Paul (30 South Fairview)	(612) 690-0197

MISSOURI

Wild Oats Community Market

Kansas City (4301 Main St.)	(816) 931-1873
St. Louis (8823 Ladue Rd.)	(314) 721-8004

NEW JERSEY

Fresh Fields

Millburn (187 Millburn Ave.)	(201) 376-4668
Montclair (701 Bloomfield Ave.)	(201) 746-5110

NEW MEXICO

Alfalfa's Market

Santa Fe (333 W. Cordova Rd.)	(505) 986-8667

Wild Oats Community Market

Albequerque (6300 A San Mateo NE)	(505) 823-1933
Albequerque (11015 Menaul Blvd. NE)	(505) 275-6660
Santa Fe (1090 St. Francis Dr.)	(505) 983-5333
Santa Fe (1708 Llano St.)	(505) 473-4943

NEVADA

Wild Oats Community Market

Las Vegas (3455 E. Flamingo)	(702) 434-8115
Las Vegas (6720 W. Sahara)	(702) 253-7050

NEW YORK

Fresh Fields

Munsey Park (2101 Northern Blvd.)	(516) 869-8900

NORTH CAROLINA

Wellspring Grocery

Durham (621 Broad St.)	(919) 286-0371
Raleigh (3540 Wade Ave.)	(919) 828-5805

Whole Foods Market

Chapel Hill (81 South Elliot)	(919) 968-1983

OREGON

Oasis Market

Eugene (2489 Willamette St.)	(541) 345-1014
Eugene (2580 Willakenzie)	(541) 334-6382

PENNSYLVANIA

Fresh Fields

North Wales (1210 Bethlehem Pike)	(215) 646-6300
Philadelphia (2001 Pennsylvania Ave.)	(215) 557-0015
Wynnewood (339 East Lancaster Ave.)	(610) 896-3737

Whole Foods Market

Wayne (821 Lancaster Ave.)	(610) 688-9400

RHODE ISLAND

Whole Foods Market

Providence (261 Waterman St.)	(401) 272-1690

TENNESSEE

Wild Oats Community Market

Memphis (5101 Sanderlin)	(901) 685-2293
Memphis (1801 Union Ave.)	(901) 725-4823

Sunshine Grocery

Nashville (3201 Belmont Blvd.)	(615) 297-5100

TEXAS

Whole Foods Market

Austin (601 North Lamar, Suite 100)	(512) 476-1206
Austin (9607 Research Blvd., #300)	(512) 345-5003
Dallas (7205 Skillman St.)	(214) 341-5445
Houston (2900 S. Shepherd.)	(713) 520-1937
Plano (2201 Preston Rd., Suite C)	(972) 612-6729
Richardson (60 Dal-Rich Village)	(972) 699-8075
San Antonio (255 E. Basse Rd., Ste 130)	(210) 826-4676

UTAH

Wild Oats Community Market

Salt Lake City (812 E. 200 South)	(801) 355-7401

VIRGINIA

Fresh Fields

Alexandria (6548 Little River Turnpike)	(703) 914-0040
Arlington (2700 Wilson Blvd.)	(703) 527-6596
Vienna (143 Maple Avenue East)	(703) 319-2000
Falls Church (7511 Leesburg Pike)	(703) 448-1600
Reston (11660 Plaza America Dr.)	(703) 736-0600
Springfield (8402 Old Keene Mill Rd.)	(703) 644-2500

Whole Foods Market

Charlottesville (1416 Seminole Trail)	(804) 973-4900

WASHINGTON, D.C.

Whole Foods Market

Georgetown (2323 Wisconsin Ave.)	(202) 333-5393

Fresh Fields

Tenley Circle (4630 40th Street, NW)	(202) 237-5800

WISCONSIN

Whole Foods Market

Madison (3313 University Ave.)	(608) 233-9566

CANADA (BRITISH COLUMIBIA)

Wild Oats Community Market

Vancouver (2285 West 4th Ave.)	(604) 739-6676
West Vancouver (2496 Marine Dr.)	(604) 925-3316

Low-Fat and Low-Calorie Baking

Some of the most common drugs used to treat interstitial cystitis have weight gain as a side effect. As a result, many of us have to carefully watch our fat and calorie intake. You may also have other medical reasons for wanting to adjust the fat and calorie content of favorite recipes. Or perhaps you've thought of making up your own recipes to fit your medical situation, but weren't feeling confident of your cooking skills.

Baked goods are probably the hardest to improvise, because they are dependent on complex reactions of a number of ingredients. Here are some tips for altering or inventing recipes for baked goods:

◆ Cholesterol

You can lower the cholesterol by using two egg whites in place of each whole egg in most quick breads, cookies, and cakes. (Yes, this actually works!)

◆ Fats

Fats contribute to the tenderness of baked goods so you have to be careful in lowering the amount. To lower the amount of fat in baked goods, use lowfat (1 percent or 2 percent) or skim milk when milk is called for in items like cookies, cakes, and breads. The minimum amount of fat for muffins, quick breads, and biscuits is 1 to 2 tablespoons per cup of flour. Any less will detract from the tenderness. Some yeast breads (such as English muffins or french bread) can be made with no fat. Cakes however, need a little fat to keep them moist and tender. About 2 Tbsp. per cup of flour is a minimum. As for cookies, drop cookies are usually softer and generally contain less fat than crisp rolled cookies. The fat level for rolled cookies can usually be adjusted to 2 tablespoons per cup of flour. Lowering the fat too much in rolled cookies can make a dough that is tough and difficult to roll out.

◆ Sugar

Sugars contribute flavor and also affect the tenderness and volume of baked products. Add a bit more spice to baked products to enhance the flavor if you reduce the sugar or other sweeteners. In general, use half a cup of sugar per cup of flour in cakes. (Using less sugar will make the cake more like a quick bread). For muffins and quick breads, the ratio is usually 1 Tbsp. sugar per cup of flour. In yeast breads, only use a teaspoon of sugar per cup of flour.

A Word About Ethylene Gas

When fruit ripens naturally on the plant it slowly converts the acids to sugars as the fruit becomes ripe. Unfortunately, commercial growers pick fruit while it is still firm and slightly green to prevent damage in shipping. This is true for almost all fruit, including tomatoes.

The public however, is not likely to buy a green tomato or apricot at the store, so the fruit is treated with ethylene gas to "ripen" it. Ethylene gas is naturally given off by flowers and ripening fruit. When green fruit is exposed to ethylene gas, the rind or skin turns color and the fruit begins to age. (But the gas doesn't make an utterly green fruit ripen exactly as it would on the plant— hence the red but pithy cardboard tomatoes, and the tasteless, crunchy, but thoroughly yellow apricots).

At home, you can use fruit's natural ethylene gas to your advantage to speed the ripening of pears, or other fruit that you may be able to eat. Just put them in a paper bag and tie the end shut. If you include a banana (a notorious ethylene gas producer), the process will go faster. Have you seen the "banana hangers"— hooks that suspend a bunch of bananas above a tabletop? Increased air circulation helps bananas last longer than they would in a fruit bowl. (According to Dr. Devin Starlanyl, slightly green bananas may have less bladder-irritating tyramine, too).

There are two IC-friendly fruits that can be picked green and will ripen without being "gassed"— pears and honeydew melons. After being picked green, they continue to convert their acids to sugar, actually ripening, not just getting old. You can spot a very ripe honeydew melon because the rind will be slightly sticky with fruit sugar. (Unless the store has washed them off).

Although the flowers on the dinner table aren't for eating, they too get old and turn brown when exposed to ethylene gas. Because flowers also naturally produce ethylene gas, florists who store them in coolers need to be concerned about gas build up that ages the flowers faster, making them wilt and turn brown. Nothing is worse for fresh flowers than to be stored overnight in the fruit-filled produce cooler of a supermarket.

Some vegetables, such as lettuce, are exceedingly sensitive to ethylene gas. At home, you can have the same problem in your refrigerator that florists do in their coolers. For long lasting fresh vegetables, don't store gas-producing fruit and tomatoes in a small closed compartment with your lettuce and other salad vegetables. Remember too, that as fruits go from ripe to spoiled they can become high in tyramine. If you are particularly sensitive to tyramine, you may find that overripe or slightly spoiled foods can bother your bladder even if those foods are usually okay for you to eat.

Safe Preservation of Low-Acid Foods

Home canning and freezing are two ways to preserve store bought or home-grown food for later use. Processing the food correctly is important both for the taste and appearance of the product, and its safety.

Canning

The canning process is designed to preserve food by heating it enough to destroy spoilage causing organisms. Once the food is heated and the organisms killed, the containers must be sealed to prevent the food from becoming contaminated. Safe canning depends on three variables: acidity, time, and temperature.

For high-acid foods like pickles, jellies, and fruits, a water-bath canner is used. In this process boiling water in an open kettle heats the jars to the temperature of boiling water— 212° F. That is sufficient for high-acid foods because the acid helps keep the bacteria level in check, but it is not a safe procedure for low-acid foods.

Tomatoes have always been thought to be acid enough to be canned safely by the water-bath method— without a pressure canner or added acid. In the past, because of tomatoes' acidity, the USDA hasn't encouraged people to use a pressure canner for them. Very recently, however, it was discovered that some bacteria can grow at the acid level of tomatoes, so the USDA is beginning to rethink their advice. They have recently issued new guidelines for canning tomatoes, which advise people to add lemon juice or citric acid to tomatoes they home-can by the water-bath method.

For low-acid foods, such as those we eat on an IC diet, the temperature of boiling water is not sufficient to insure food safety. Meats, vegetables, and fish must be processed in a pressure canner where increased pressure boosts temperatures into the 220° F. to 250° F. range. If you grow low-acid tomatoes at home and plan on canning them, it would probably be wise to consider pressure-canning them, too. The USDA considers it safe to can low-acid foods in a pressure canner, without adding acid. (Years ago I used a pressure-canner to can chopped tomatoes as if they were meat. It was my first canning experience and I over-processed them enormously. The chunks of tomato fell apart as a result of the lengthy cooking, but they tasted just wonderful when I used them in home-made soups).

The U.S. Department of Agriculture in cooperation with many universities, publishes guidelines for home canning and freezing of fruits and vegetables. Your phone directory should list a number for your local university's cooperative extension office. If there isn't one near you, the University of California Division of Agriculture and Natural Resources has some good inexpensive booklets on safe home canning and freezing procedures, which gives the times needed to safely process various foods. They can be ordered by phone at (510) 642-2431 using a credit card. Listed below are three titles and their cost. You can also order these booklets by enclosing a check for the cost of each booklet plus one dollar for shipping and handling. Send order to: ANR Publications, University of California, 6701 San Pablo Ave.,Oakland, CA 94608. (It usually takes two weeks to get the booklets, and they ask that you indicate the booklet numbers on your order).

#21392 Home Canning of Fruits and Vegetables (12 pages) $1.75

#2725 Home Freezing of Meats, Poultry, Fish and Shellfish (12 pages) $1.75

#2724 Home Freezing of Vegetables (16 pages) $1.75

Here's another safety tip from the food experts at the U.S. Department of Agriculture. If you can meats and vegetables, never taste these low-acid foods cold from the jar. (For low-acid tomatoes, it would probably be wise to follow the same principle). Cook them for 10 or 20 minutes first, before tasting. Harmful toxins from certain bacteria may not change the appearance or smell of the food. If in doubt when you open the jar, don't use it.

Freezing

Freezing is another way to preserve food. It's quicker to do and less messy than canning, but you can use up all your refrigerator's freezer space quickly if you freeze very much. Consider the costs-versus-benefits of a separate freezer. You may find that the reduced number of bladder-bouncing trips to the store and convenience of quick meal preparation are worth the cost.

If you have a separate freezer, a freezer thermometer is a good investment. I've used an Eddie Bauer ski thermometer— it hangs from a convenient clip which was originally designed to attach to a jacket zipper. It's small, easy to move around, and never falls off the freezer rack.

Keep the temperature of your separate freezer lower than that of your refrigerator freezer. The U.S. Department of Agriculture and the University of California Division of Agricultural Sciences both advise a temperature of 0 degrees F. or below. (I found out the hard way though, that keeping your refrigerator's freezer very cold is not a good idea. My favorite vanilla ice cream was too rock hard to eat). Colder temperatures slow down the enzymes that deteriorate food. As the storage temperature increases above 0° F., the length of time you can store food decreases. For instance, a vegetable that maintains flavor and texture for a year at 0° F., will start to lose quality after only three months at 10° F., and will deteriorate after 3 weeks at 20° F. Make sure food is fresh and not old or contaminated before freezing. Freezing won't kill bacteria.

Most vegetables freeze well but some don't. These don't freeze well: radishes, lettuce, green onions and some whole tomatoes. If you want to freeze your home-grown low-acid tomatoes, try making juice out of them, making tomato sauce, or using them in a soup, stew, or casserole. In my experience, whole, ripe, low-acid tomatoes fall apart and get mushy.

MEASURES ...

1 quart = 2 pints = 4 cups = 0.946 liters

1 cup = 8 fluid ounces = 1/2 pint = 16 tablespoons

1/4 cup = 4 tablespoons

1 tablespoon = 3 teaspoons

1 cup fine graham cracker crumbs = 14 square graham crackers

1 cup fine cracker crumbs = 28 square saltine crackers

1 cup whipped cream = 1/2 cup whipping cream

1 clove garlic = 1/8 tsp dry garlic powder

1 cup of soft bread crumbs = 1-1/2 slices of bread

1 cup chopped pears = 1 whole pear

1 cup cooked rice = 1/2 cup dry rice

...AND SUBSTITUTIONS

For thickening: 1 Tbsp. cornstarch = 2 Tbsp. flour = 1 Tbsp. potato flour = 4 tsp. dry tapioca.

For sweetening: 1 cup sugar = 7/8 cup honey = 1 cup maple syrup plus 1/4 cup corn syrup.

For corn syrup: 1 cup corn syrup = 1-3/4 cup sugar plus 1/3 cup liquid.

For cake flour: 1 cup cake flour = 1 cup minus 2 Tbsp. all-purpose flour.

For baking powder: 1 tsp. baking powder = 1/2 tsp. cream of tartar plus 1/4 tsp. baking soda, plus 1/4 tsp. cornstarch (or 1/4 tsp. flour if you are allergic to corn).

For chocolate: 1 Tbsp. carob powder can be substituted for 1 Tbsp. of cocoa powder. In recipes calling for unsweetened baking chocolate squares, try using 3 Tbsp. carob powder plus 1 Tbsp. butter or margarine for each 1-ounce square of unsweetened chocolate.

For cloves: Try using equal amounts of powdered allspice for powdered cloves in baked goods, desserts, and marinades.

For dried parsley: Try using equal amounts of dried chervil.

For Worcestershire sauce: In cooking, try using equal parts allspice and onion salt.

APPENDIX C

Organizations and Other Resources

These organizations have been very helpful to many people with IC and other IC-associated disorders. Don't hesitate to contact them with questions or concerns—they are there to help.

Interstitial Cystitis Association (ICA)
P.O. Box 1553
Madison Square Station
New York, NY 10159-1553

phone: (212) 979-6057

Pamphlets, tapes, videos and educational materials are available ($1 to $17.50, with most in the $3 to $5 range). Quarterly newsletter for $40 contribution. Referrals to local support groups and urologists, telephone support network.

Canadian Interstitial Cystitis Society (CICS)
P.O. Box 28625
406 S. Willingdon Ave.
Burnaby, B.C.
V5C 6J4

phone: (250) 758-3207
FAX: (250) 758-4894

Membership organization ($35.00/yr). Provides telephone network, educational materials, referrals to local groups, quarterly newsletter.

Fibromyalgia Network
P.O. Box 31750
Tucson, AZ 85751-1750

phone: (520) 290-5508
FAX: (520) 290-5550

Quarterly newsletter ($19.00/yr). Referrals to local chapters, educational information available, free information packet on request.

Arthritis Foundation
P.O. Box 7669
Atlanta, GA 30357-0669

phone: (800) 933-0032 or
phone: (800) 283-7800

Educational material on fibromyalgia, osteoarthritis, and rheumatoid arthritis, referrals to local chapters and offices, exercise classes, free brochures on request, magazine (6 issues/ yr.) with membership ($20 per year).

International Foundation for Functional Gastrointestinal Disorders (IFFGD)
P.O. Box 17864
Milwaukee, WI 53217

phone: (414) 964-1799 or
(888) 964-2001 (toll free)
FAX: (414) 964-7176

Quarterly newsletter for members ($25.00/yr). Educational materials on irritable bowel syndrome (IBS), colitis, pelvic floor pain, GERD, and many other gastrointestinal conditions.

IBS Self Help Group
3332 Yonge Street
P.O. Box 94074
Toronto, Ontario
Canada M4N 3R1

Membership organization, suggested donation, $15.00. Provides information on irritable bowel syndrome to patients, referrals to local groups.

National Digestive Diseases Information Clearinghouse
2 Information Way
Bethesda, MD 20892-3570

phone: (301) 654-3810

Part of National Institutes of Health (NIH), under U.S. Public Health Service. Provides information to patients about irritable bowel syndrome and other conditions.

National Vulvodynia Association (NVA)
P.O. Box 4491
Silver Spring, MD 20914-4491

phone: (301) 299-0775
FAX: (301) 299-3999

Educational materials, referrals to local support, quarterly newsletter ($35.00/yr.), patient-to-patient support.

Vulvar Pain Foundation (VPF)
P. O. Drawer 177
Graham, NC 27253

phone: (910) 226-0704 (Tues. & Thurs)
FAX: (910) 226-8518

Referrals to local support groups, quarterly newsletter, Low-oxalate diet cookbook available.

National Headache Foundation
428 W. St. James Place, 2nd Floor
Chicago, IL 60614-2750

phone: (800) 843-2256 (toll free)
FAX: (773) 525-7357

Free migraine educational materials. Audio/video tapes and brochures, available. Referrals to support groups nationwide. List of physician members. Quarterly newsletter with membership, ($20/ yr).

American Academy of Allergy, Asthma & Immunology
611 East Wells Street
Milwaukee, WI 53202-3889

phone: (414) 272-6071 or
(800) 822-2762 (toll free)

Educational pamphlets for patients on allergies, asthma, and related problems including food allergy and food intolerances. (One pamphlet each subject, free. Call for price of multiple copies).

American Pain Society and **American Academy of Pain Medicine**
4700 W. Lake Ave.
Glenview, IL 60025

phone: (847) 375-4715
FAX: (847) 375-4777

Information on pain management and pain medications, list of pain clinics by state and type of services. (Their consensus statement, *The Use of Opioids for the Treatment of Chronic Pain* is helpful when talking with doctors about pain management strategies).

American Dietetic Association
P. O. Box 97215
Chicago, IL 60678-7215

phone: (800) 366-1655

Educational materials on gluten intolerance, food allergy, lactose intolerance, and others. Referrals to local registered dieticians, state dietetic organizations. For per/minute fee, callers can talk to registered dietician, (900) 225-5267.

Electronic/Internet Resources

For those who have a computer at home or work and access to the Internet, a wealth of information and emotional support resources are available. But be careful—just as the Internet is a great conduit of information just waiting to be tapped, it can also be a great conduit for misinformation, scam artists, and patient exploitation. Before trying anything new, it is a good idea to check out what you find with your doctor.

Websites and E-mail Addresses

There are many, many sources of information on IC and IC-related disorders available through the Internet— far too many to mention here. A search engine such as Webcrawler or Yahoo (http://www.yahoo.com) can come up with plenty of excellent IC-related sites. You'll be surprised at the sheer number of traditional and alternative medical approaches that exist. Although not an exhaustive listing, the few websites below are a good start in your quest for information. (Web addresses change frequently, so if you can't connect, try a search for the site name with a search engine).

IC Network (ICN)	http://www.sonic.net/jill/icnet/	(old)
	http://www.ic-network.com	(new)
Interstitial Cystitis Association (ICA)	http://www.ichelp.org	
Canadian Interstitial Cystitis Society (CICS)	http://www.sonic.net/jill/icnet/canada	
International Foundation for Functional Gastrointestinal Disorders (IFFGD)	http://www.iffgd.org	
IBS Self Help Group	http://www.ibsgroup.org	
Mediconsult (links to sites for various diseases)	http://www.mediconsult.com	
National Headache Foundation	http://www.HEADACHES.org	

Neurologist online (headaches, pain issues)	http://www.eastnc2.coastalnet.com/~cn3877/
Arthritis Foundation	http://www.arthritis.org
Dr. Starlanyl's Fibromyalgia and Myofascial Pain Syndrome Page	http://www.sover.net/~devstar
Fibromyalgia Network	http://www.fmnetnews.com
Oregon Fibromyalgia Foundation	http://www.myalgia.com
National Vulvodynia Association (NVA)	http://www.nva.org
American Pain Society	http://www.ampainsoc.org
Pharmaceutical Information Network	http://www.pharminfo.com

Newsgroups, Chat Rooms and Message Boards

There's nothing like talking to someone who's been there and knows what you're going through. The community of people with IC extends worldwide, and is becoming connected via the Internet. The perfect medium for those whose urinary frequency makes it difficult to get out of the house, the Internet has several places where IC patients meet and exchange messages.

Some Internet message boards are moderated, so that unwanted pornographic or commercial messages are filtered out, while others are totally uncensored and "anything goes." The unmoderated boards are occasionally clogged with "spam" (unsolicited advertisements and pornographic messages), and not for the easily offended. Nonetheless these message boards are accessible to a growing group of IC patients in many countries. Often the first contact that an IC patient has with others who share the difficulties of chronic illness is through these message boards. Many touching stories and informative messages are exchanged daily at the places listed below. If you are new to both IC and the Internet, you may want to just "lurk" (read the messages without posting any yourself) for awhile until you get the hang of it. Happy surfing on the net!

America Online IC Support Group ***(moderated)***	Meets on alternate Wednesday evenings at 6:30 pm PT (9:30 pm ET), in private chat room "IC Support Group".
America Online Message Boards ***(moderated)***	***For IC:*** At Keyword, type in "dis". Choose "Message Boards", choose "Kidney & Urinary Tract Disorders", scroll to Interstitial Cystitis. ***For IBS:*** At Keyword, type in "dis" Choose "Message Boards". choose "Abdomen and Digestive Disorders", scroll to Irritable Bowel Syndrome.
IC Network Message Boards and Chat ***(moderated)***	See the ICN website for up-to-date details. The IC Network has the most extensive and inclusive group of moderated IC message boards and is continually in a process of upgrading and expanding. There are boards for everyone with IC, as well as more specific ones for men with IC, for spouses of IC patients, for Christians with IC, and one dedicated to the topic of sexuality and IC.
Interstitial Cystitis Newsgroup ***(unmoderated)***	alt.support.inter-cystitis
Prostatitis Newsgroup (helpful for men with IC) ***(unmoderated)***	sci.med.prostatitis
Migraine Newsgroup ***(unmoderated)***	alt.support.headaches.migraine
Fibromyalgia Newsgroup ***(unmoderated)***	alt.med.fibromyalgia
Irritable Bowel Syndrome Newsgroup ***(unmoderated)***	alt.support.ibs

APPENDIX D

For Further Reading

Chronic pain:

Freedom from Pain, N. J. Marcus, M.D. and J.S. Arbeiter, 1994, Simon & Schuster.

Living with Chronic Illness, Days of Patience and Passion, Cheri Register, 1992, Bantam

Relieving Pain (pamphlet), National Institutes of Health, Office of Clinical Center Communications (single copies available from: NIH/OCCC, Relieving Pain/IC, Building 10, Room 1C255, 9000 Rockville Pike, Bethesda , MD 20892).

Sick and Tired of Feeling Sick and Tired: living with invisible chronic illness, Paul J. Donoghue PhD., and Mark E. Siegel, PhD., 1992, Norton.

We Are Not Alone- Learning to Live with Chronic Illness, Sefra Kobrin Pitzele, 1986 Workman Publishing.

Fibromyalgia:

Conquering Carpal Tunnel Syndrome and other Repetitive Strain Injuries, Sharon Butler, 1995, Advanced Press.

Fibromyalgia & Chronic Myofascial Pain Syndrome- A survival manual, Devin Starlanyl, M.D. and M.E. Copeland, M.S., M.A., 1996, New Harbinger Publications.

Getting to Sleep, Ellen Mohr Catelano, 1990, New Harbinger Publications, Oakland, CA.

Interstitial Cystitis, General Bladder Disorders:

Overcoming Bladder Disorders, R. Chalker and K.E. Whitmore, M.D., 1990, Harper Row.

Irritable Bowel Syndrome:

Learning to Live with Chronic IBS: a practical guide to irritable bowel syndrome, N. Tannenhaus, 1990, Dell Publishing.

Relief From IBS, E. Shimberg, 1988, Evans and Co.

The Wellness Book of IBS, D. Scanlon and B. Bechel, 1989, St. Martin's Press.

Migraine and Other Headaches:

Migraine, Oliver Sacks, 1992, University of California Press.

The Hormone Headache, S. Diamond, M.D., B. Still, and C. Still, (219 pages, available through the National Headache Foundation).

Sexuality:

Seven Weeks to Better Sex, D. Renshaw, M.D., 1995, American Medical Association.

Enabling Romance: A Guide to Love, Sex, and Relationships for the Disabled and the People Who Care About Them, call the Special Needs Project at (888) 333-6867 for a booklist which includes this and other titles.

Special Diets and Cookbooks:

Headache and Diet: Tyramine-free recipes, S. Diamond, M.D., D. Francis, A.D. Vye (173 pages, available through the National Headache Foundation).

The Low-Oxalate Cookbook, (available through the Vulvar Pain Foundation).

Irritable Bowel Syndrome: Special Diet Cookbooks, A. Page-Wood and J. Davies, 1991, Thorsons.

The Allergy Self-Help Cookbook, Marjorie Hurt Jones, R.N., 1984, Rodale Press, Emmaus, Pennsylvania. (Hard to find in small bookstores. Public libraries often have it).

APPENDIX E

Vegetarian Recipe Index

✿ Appetizers

✿ Bread and Breakfast

✿ Cakes and Frostings

✿ Cookies

✿ Lunches and Snacks

✿ Meat and Main Dishes

✿ Pies and Desserts

✿ Soups and Stews

✿ Vegetables, Salads and Side Dishes

✿ Miscellaneous

Low-Oxalate Recipe Index

✓ Appetizers

✓ Bread and Breakfast

✓ Cakes and Frostings

✓ Cookies

✓ Lunches and Snacks

✓ Meat and Main Dishes

✓ Pies and Desserts

✓ Seafood

✓ Soups and Stews

✓ Vegetables, Salads and Side Dishes

✓ Miscellaneous

BIBLIOGRAPHY

Abu-Arafeh, I. and G. Russell. 1995. Prevalance and clinical features of abdominal migraine compared with those of migraine headache. *Archives of Disease in Childhood,* 72 (5): 413-417.

Alagiri, M., S. Chottiner, et. al. 1997. Interstitial cystitis: unexplained associations with other chronic disease and pain syndromes. *Urology,* 49 (supp. 5A).

All About Vegetables. 1990. Ortho Books, 200 Bush Street San Francisco, CA 94104

Amerine, Maynard A. and Vernon L. Singleton. 1977. *Wine: An introduction,* 2nd ed. University of California Press.

American Academy of Allergy, Asthma, and Immunology. 1995. *Adverse Reactions to Food Additives.* 611 E. Wells St., Milwaukee, WI 53202-3889

Antioxidants for athletes. 1995. *University of California Berkeley Wellness Letter.* 11 (4).

Appenzeller, O. 1991. Pathogenesis of migraine. *Medical Clinics of North America,* 75 (3): 763-789.

Bear, John and Marina Bear. 1987. *How to Repair Food.* Berkeley, CA. Ten Speed Press.

Berkoff, Nancy. March 6, 1997. Weekly Produce Report. *Orange County Register.* Santa Ana, CA.

Beshadri, P., Emerson L., et al. 1994. Cimetidine in the treatment of interstitial cystitis. *Urology,* 44.

Birder, L.A., A.J. Kanai, and W.C. deGroat. 1997. DMSO: Effect on bladder afferent neurons and nitric oxide release. *Journal of Urology,* 158 (5), 1989-1995.

Blackwell, Barry, M.D. No date. *Are you a gut responder? Hints on coping with an irritable bowel.* International Foundation for Functional Gastrointestinal Disorders. P.O. Box 17864, Milwaukee, WI 53217.

Bladder Retraining Reduces Urinary Frequency. 1996. *ICA Update,* 11 (1): 2. Interstitial Cystitis Association, P.O. Box 1553, Madison Square Station, New York, NY 10159.

Block, Zenas. 1981. *It's All on the Label: understanding food additives and nutrition.* Little Brown & Co.

Cinnabon (commercial informational pamphlet). 1997. Cinnabon Company. Seattle Washington.

Clauw, Daniel, M.D. 1995. Fibromyalgia: more than just a musculoskeletal disease. *American Family Physician,* 52 (3).

Dalessio, Donald J., M.D. 1991. *Migraine: information for patients.* Organon Inc.

Davids, Kenneth. 1991. *Coffee: A Guide to Buying, Brewing, and Enjoying.* 101Productions. Santa Rosa, CA.

Diedrich Coffee (commercial informational pamphlet). 1997. Diedrich Coffee, Inc. Irvine, CA.

Dixon, J.S. and T. Hald. Morphological Studies of the Bladder Wall in Interstitial Cystitis. *Sensory Disorders of the Bladder and Urethra.* 1986. Edited by N.J.R. George and J.A. Gosling. Berlin. Springer-Verlag.

Dudek, Susan G. 1997. *Nutrition Handbook for Nursing Practice,* 3rd edition. Phildelphia, PA. Lippincott-Raven.

Eisenburg, Arlene and Heidi Murkoff. 1984. How to Read a Food Label. *American Health,* (July-Aug).

Elbadawi, Ahmad. 1997. Interstitial cystitis: a critique of current concepts with a new proposal for pathologic diagnosis and pathogenesis. *Urology,* 49 (supp 5A).

Elkort, Martin Edward. 1991. *The secret life of food: a feast of food and drink history, folklore and fact.* New York, NY. St. Martin's Press.

Foods and Nutrition Encyclopedia. 1983. Edited by Audrey H.Ensminger, M. E. Ensminger, James E. Konlande and John R.K. Robson, M.D.. Pegus Press.

Garey, Terry. 1996. *The Joy of Home Winemaking.* New York, NY. Avon Books.

Goldenberg, Don L., M.D. 1995. *Fibromyalgia Syndrome.* Arthritis Foundation.

Goodman, Harriet Willinsky and Barbara Morse. 1982. *Just What the Doctor Ordered.* New York, NY. Holt, Rinehart and Winston.

Handbook of Food Additives, 2nd ed. 1972. Edited by Thomas Furia. CRC Press.

Heartburn relief: the acid test. 1997. *University of California Berkeley Wellness Letter.* 14 (1).

Heaton, Kenneth W., M.D. 1997. Diet and Functional Bowel Disease. *Participate,* 6 (1). International Foundation for Functional Gastrointestinal Disorders. P.O. Box 17864, Milwaukee, WI 53217.

Herbst, Sharon Tyler. *The Food Lover's Companion,* 2nd ed. 1997. Barron's Educational Services.

Hillman, Howard. 1989. *Kitchen Science.* New York, NY. Houghton-Mifflin.

Hoag Hospital Emergency Department, (Newport Beach , CA). No date. *Bland Diet* (patient information sheet).

Horticultural Data Processors. 1995. *Avant Gardener,* 28 (3). New York, NY.

How powerful is Pycnogenol? 1997. *University of California Berkeley Wellness Letter.* 14 (2).

Illy, Francesco and Ricardo Illy. 1992. *The Book of Coffee.* Abbeville Press. New York, NY.

Introduction to Chemical Principles. 1983. Edited by H. Stephen Stoker. New York, NY. Macmillan.

Irritable Bowel Syndrome (IBS). 1993. International Foundation for Functional Gastrointestinal Disorders. P.O. Box 17864, Milwaukee, WI 53217.

Johnson, Elaine. 1997. The sweeter side of Meyer lemons. *Sunset,* (March).

Jones, Marjorie Hurt, R.N. 1984. *The Allergy Self-Help Cookbook.* Emmaus, PA. Rodale Press.

Jones, C.A. and L. Nyberg. 1997. Epidemiology of Interstitial Cystitis. *Urology,* 49 (supp. 5A).

Keay, S., C.-O. Zhang, D.I. Kagen, M.K. Hise, et al. 1997. Concentrations of specific epithelial growth factors in the urine of interstitial cystitis patients and controls. *Journal of Urology,* 158(5), 1983-1988.

Koziol, J.A., D.C. Clark, R.F. Gittes, E. M. Tan. 1993. The natural history of interstitial cystitis: a survey of 374 patients. *Journal of Urology,* 149: 465-469.

Kreiter, Ted. 1995. A Microbiologist Who Stopped Her Fever Blisters. *Saturday Evening Post,* (Nov/Dec).

Laguna Hills Nursery, (Geronimo Road, Lake Forest, CA.). no date. *Tropical and Subtropical Fruits* (fact sheet).

L-Arginine Reduces IC Pain in Preliminary Study. 1996. *ICA Update,* 11 (2): 7. Interstitial Cystitis Association, P.O. Box 1553, Madison Square Station, New York, NY 10159.

Larousse Gastronomique. 1984. Edited by J. H. Lang. New York, NY. Crown Publishers.

Lewi, Henry M.D., F.R.C.S. (Dept. of Urology, Broomfield Hospital, U.K.). 1995. Cimetidine in treatment of interstitial cystitis. letter. *Urology,* 45 (6): 1088.

MacNeil, Karen. 1981. *The Book of Whole Foods: Nutrition and cuisine.* New York, NY. Random House.

Marinoff, S.C. and M.L.C. Turner. 1992. Vulvar Vestibulitis Syndrome. *Dermatologic Clinics,* 10(2).

McCarthy, Ed and Mary Ewing-Mulligan. 1997. *White Wine for Dummies.* IDG Books Worldwide, Inc.

McKay, Marilyn. 1992. Vulvodynia: diagnostic patterns. *Dermatologic Clinics,* 10.

Merck Manual, 16th edition. 1992. Edited by Robert Berkow, M.D., Andrew J. Fletcher, M.D., et al. Whitehouse Station, NJ. Merck & Co., Inc.

Mirkin, Gabriel, M.D. 1996. *Foods and Migraine, report #6760.* Mirkin Report. Internet website. http://www.wdn.com/mirkin

Nachel, Marty and Steve Ettinger. 1996. *Beer for Dummies.* IDG Books Worldwide, Inc.

National Vulvodynia Association. 1995. *NVA News,* 1(1). P.O. Box 9309, Silver Spring, MD 20906-9309.

Nettleton, Joyce, D.Sc., R.D. 1985, (rev.1987). *Seafood and Health.* Osprey Books.

Nicolodi, M. and F. Sicuteri. 1996. Fibromyalgia and migraine, two faces of the same mechanism. Serotonin as the common clue for pathogenesis and therapy. *Advances in Experimental Medicine and Biology,* 398: 373-379.

Nye, David, M.D. 1997. *Fibromyalgia: A Guide for Patients.* Internet website. nyeda@uwec.edu

Onions. *Epicurious.* Internet website. http://www.epicurious.com (March 1997).

Paganelli, R., U. Fagiolo, M. Cancian, G.C. Sturniolo, E. Scala, and G.P. D'Offizi. Intestinal permeability in irritable bowel syndrome. Effect of diet and sodium cromoglycate administration. 1990. *Annals of Allergy*, Volume 64: 377-379.

Parsons, C. Lowell, M.D. 1996. Doctor's Forum. *ICA Update,* 11 (3): 4-5. Interstitial Cystitis Association, P.O. Box 1553, Madison Square Station, New York, NY 10159.

Potera, Carol. 1996. Prozac of the Sea. *Psychology Today.* (May/June).

Reavis, Charles G. 1995. *Home Sausage Making.* Storey Communications. Pownal, VT.

Recommended Dietary Allowances, 9th ed. 1980. National Academy of Sciences.

Reuters Health Information Services. 1996. Cimetidine shows efficacy in Treatment of Interstitial Cystitis Symptoms. *Reuters Medical News.* Paris, France. Internet website, (Sept. 9). http://www.reutershealth.com

Rosenthal, Sylvia and Fran Shinagel. 1981. *How Cooking Works.* New York, NY. Macmillan.

Sacks, Oliver, M.D. 1992. *Migraine.* Los Angeles, CA. University of California Press.

Salzman, A.L. 1995. Nitric oxide in the gut. *New Horizons*, 3 (2): 352-364.

Sandler, M., N.Y. Li, N. Jarrett, V. Glover. 1995. Dietary migraine: recent progress in the red (and white) wine story. *Cephalagia*, 15 (2): 101-103.

Saper, Joel R., M.D., F.A.C.P. 1987. *Help for Headaches.* (adapted from Headache Disorders). New York, NY. Warner.

Scher, W., and B. M. Scher. 1992. A possible role for nitric oxide in glutamate (MSG)-induced Chinese restaurant syndrome, glutamate-induced asthma, 'hot-dog headache', pugilistic Alzheimer's disease, and other disorders. *Medical Hypotheses*, 38(2), 185-188.

Sears, Barry, PhD. 1995. *The Zone: a dietary road map.* Harper-Collins.

Shaudys, Phyllis V. 1986. *The Pleasure of Herbs.* Storey Communications. Pownal, VT.

Similarities Between IC, Inflammatory Bowel Disease, and Irritable Bowel Syndrome. 1996. *ICA Update,* 11 (4): 9. Interstitial Cystitis Association, P.O. Box 1553, Madison Square Station, New York, NY 10159.

Smith, Shannon D., Marcia A. Wheeler, Harris E. Foster, Jr., et al. 1996. Urinary Nitric Oxide Synthase Activity and Cyclic GMP Levels are Decreased with Interstitial Cystitis and Increased with Urinary Tract Infections. *Journal of Urology,* 155: 1432-1435.

Spanos, C., X. Pang, K. Ligris, et al. 1997. Stress-induced bladder mast cell activation: implications for interstitial cystitis. *Journal of Urology,* 157: 669-672.

Starlanyl, Devin, M.D. and Mary Ellen Copeland. 1996. *Fibromyalgia and Chronic Myofascial Pain Syndrome: a survival manual.* Oakland, CA. New Harbinger Publications.

Stauth, Cameron. 1995. Beating Chronic Fatigue. *Saturday Evening Post,* (Nov/Dec).

Stuckey, Maggie. 1997. *The Complete Spice Book.* New York, NY. St. Martin's Press.

The antioxidant all-stars. 1997. *University of California Berkeley Wellness Letter.* 13 (6).

The Herb Companion, 9 (3). 1997. Interweave Press, 201 E. Fourth St., Loveland CO, 80537-5655.

Theoharides, T.C. and G.R. Sant. 1997. Hydroxyzine therapy for interstitial cystitis. *Urology,* 49 (supp 5A).

Theoharides, T.C., M.D. 1993. Doctor's Forum. *ICA Update,* 8 (2): 5,8. Interstitial Cystitis Association, P.O. Box 1553, Madison Square Station, New York, NY 10159.

The PDR Family Guide to Nutrition and Health. 1995. Edited by D.W. Sifton. Montvale, NJ. Medical Economics.

Tribole, Evelyn. March 6, 1997. Histamines, alcohol in red wine may trigger headaches. *Orange County Register.* Santa Ana, CA.

Tribole, Evelyn. March 6, 1997. Nutrition and Health. *Orange County Register.* Santa Ana, CA.

Turner, Maria, M.D., et al. 1997. *National Vulvodynia Association,* (patient pamphlet). National Vulvodynia Association.

UCLA Neuroenteric Disease Section. 1997. Colonic Sensitization in IBS patients. *The Inside Trak,* 1(1).

U.S. Department of Agriculture Nutrient Data Laboratory. 1997. *Food Composition Data.* Internet website. http://nal.usda.gov/fnic/foodcomp (update: 4/13/97)

van der Meer, Antonia. 1990. *Relief from Chronic Headache.* New York, NY. Dell Books and Lynn Sonberg Book Services.

Wallace, D.J. 1990. Genitourinary manifestations of fibrositis: an increased association with the female urethral syndrome. *Journal of Rheumatology,* 17: 238-239.

Wellness facts. 1997. *University of California Berkeley Wellness Letter.* 14 (2). Western Garden Book. 1995. Sunset Publishing. Menlo Park, CA, 94025.

Whitmore, Kristene, M.D. 1996. Doctor's Forum. *ICA Update,* 11 (4): 4-5. Interstitial Cystitis Association, P.O. Box 1553, Madison Square Station, New York, NY 10159.

Whitmore, Kristene, M.D. and Rebbecca Chalker. 1990. *Overcoming Bladder Disorders.* New York, NY. Harper & Row.

Wood, Rebecca. 1988. *The Whole Foods Encyclopedia.* New York, NY. Prentice-Hall.

ALPHABETICAL INDEX TO RECIPES

Appetizers

Bread and Breakfast

Cakes and Frostings

Cookies

Lunches and Snacks

Meat and Main Dishes

Pies and Desserts

Seafood

Soups and Stews

Vegetables, Salads and Side Dishes

Miscellaneous

NOTES

NOTES

NOTES

NOTES

NOTES